Teach Yourself to Read

MODERN MEDICAL CHINESE

A Step-by-Step Workbook and Guide

by BOB FLAWS

BLUE POPPY PRESS

精勤不倦，不得道聽途

可為不可為，少天資

Published by:

Blue Poppy Press
3450 Penrose Place, Suite 110
Boulder, CO 80301
(303) 447-8372

First Edition July, 1998

ISBN 0-936185-99-6
Library of Congress #98-71172

The information in this book is given in good faith. However, the author and the
publishers cannot be held responsible for any error or omission. Nor can
they be held in any way responsible for treatment given on the basis of information
contained in this book. The publishers make this information available to English
readers for scholarly and research purposes only.

The publishers do not advocate nor endorse self-medication by laypersons. Chinese
medicine is a professional medicine. Laypersons interested in availing themselves
of the treatments described in this book should seek out a
qualified professional practitioner of Chinese medicine.

COMP Designation: Original work

Printed at Johnson Printing
Cover design by Anne Rue

10, 9, 8, 7, 6, 5, 4, 3, 2, 1

Teach Yourself to Read

MODERN MEDICAL CHINESE

精勤不倦，不得道聽途

可為不可為，少天資

by Bob Flaws

Blue Poppy Press

Preface

The first person I ever studied Chinese medicine with said in his very first class that, in order to really learn Chinese medicine well, one *has* to be able to read medical Chinese. He then proceeded to teach the class how to look Chinese characters up in a Chinese-English dictionary. This teacher was so adamant about the need for Chinese medical students to read Chinese, he would not take any long-term students who had not first studied Chinese.

At the time, I was 32 years old. I could already read, to varying degrees of fluency, Latin, French, Italian, Hindi, and Tibetan. I was way too old, I thought, to begin learning another language. So, for the next several years, I studied Chinese medicine entirely from English language sources. In 1983, I went to China to study at the Shanghai College of Traditional Chinese Medicine. The classes I took there were all taught in Chinese and then simultaneously translated into English, French, and Japanese. At first I only listened in English. Then one day, the English language translator fell ill. So I attached myself for the day to the French language group. It was then that I realized that the English and French translators were not saying the same thing. This gave me a wake up call and I began listening directly to the Chinese professor, gleaning what words I could, at the same time keeping my ears cocked to both the English and French translators. Hearing the same words over and over, day after day, and seeing Chinese characters incessantly before my eyes for three months, I learned enough Chinese to order my meals, buy things, get on and off buses and trains, and to ask directions. When I came back to the United States, I probably knew a hundred Chinese words, many of them Chinese medical technical terms, and could recognize maybe three dozen Chinese characters.

The next year I went back to China to study at the Shanghai College of TCM, and again I picked up by osmosis more words and characters. I was still way too old and way too busy to actually study Chinese. During these years, whatever Chinese medicine I learned was all in translation and the quality of anything I published at that period of my career reflects that fact. During my studies at the Shang Hai Zhong Yi Xue Yuan, I became friends with one of the translators, Zhang Ting-liang. Because I was attempting to specialize in the treatment of women's diseases, I asked Mr. Zhang to pick a basic TCM gynecology textbook to translate for publication by Blue Poppy Press. In 1985, Mr. Zhang sent me a manuscript of what was to become *A Handbook of Traditional Chinese Gynecology* which I began editing for publication. At the same time, he sent the Chinese original, *Zhong Yi Fu Ke Shou Ce*. As I edited his English language manuscript, I tried to follow along in the Chinese as best I could. Usually, I could only pick out isolated words here and there. However, I often found that Mr. Zhang had not translated every single phrase or sentence. Frequently, he would leave things out that he either felt were redundant or were in classical Chinese which he could not figure out how to put into meaningful English. At other times, I was able to read enough Chinese that it seemed to me he was often paraphrasing rather than simply saying what the Chinese appeared to be saying. Nevertheless, the first Blue Poppy edition of this text only included what he had translated, and I contented myself with merely polishing his English to make it read like a native speaker.

In 1986, I went back to Shanghai to study yet again. This time, Charles Chace, more commonly known as Chip, came with me. Chip had studied acupuncture and *kanpo yaku* at the New England School of Acupuncture, and, as part of his studies, he had taken several courses in Chinese. Therefore, Chip's ability to read Chinese was far greater than mine, although I could speak better on the street. On weekends, Chip and I would often visit the Xin Hua Shu Dian (New China Bookstore) and the Shang Hai Ke Xue Shu Dian (Shanghai Science & Technology Bookstore). There, based largely on Chip's reading the titles, we both bought dozens of TCM books for literally pennies apiece. During the same sojourn at the Shang Hai Zhong Yi Xue Yuan and also prompted by Chip, I purchased at the college bookstore the Chinese language textbook for the course we were taking. From that time forward, I attempted to follow the professor along in the Chinese text at the same time as listening to the English translation.

In the next couple of years, Blue Poppy Press published several other translations done by Zhang Ting-liang. These included *Secret Shaolin Formulae for the Treatment of Traumatic Injury, The Treatment of Cancer by Integrated Chinese-Western Medicine,* and *A Handbook of Traditional Chinese Dermatology.* In each case, during the editing process, I would go over Mr. Zhang's translation with the Chinese original, thus teaching myself more and more Chinese. However, at this point in time, I still never attempted to translate anything from scratch on my own.

During the late eighties, my wife and I ran a very small school of acupuncture and *tui na.* Mr. Zhang was a student at that school and also taught a class in Chinese medical terminology and translation. At that time, Mr. Zhang and I translated and published a number of Chinese TCM journal articles and excerpts from various Chinese TCM books. I was translating more and more and Mr. Zhang was mostly just checking my work and explaining things I simply could not make sense of. At the same time, Mr. Zhang was helping Chip with various translations and giving Chip private Chinese tutorials. We tried to teach the students at our school how to read Chinese by simply working on translations. Mr. Zhang never really taught any grammar other than explaining the grammar in the translations our various classes worked on. Likewise, students only had to study vocabulary as it appeared in whatever they were translating. Two groups of our students published several translations in the *American Journal of Acupuncture.* In addition, Honora Lee Wolfe and Rose Crescenz went on to translate and publish a book of premodern acupuncture formulas, *Highlights of Ancient Acupuncture Prescriptions.*

Finally, by the time I was in my early forties, I was no longer too old to study Chinese. The more I was able to access the Chinese medical literature, the more I realized I could not credibly perform the doctoral role I had assumed without access to a doctoral level of literature. Only the smallest fraction of the Chinese TCM literature, both premodern and contemporary, is available in English, and, as I began to read more and more Chinese, I saw that a good bit of that literature is not well and accurately translated. I have been told by one Chinese scholar that there are 30,000 extant volumes of premodern Chinese literature (meaning pre-20th century). In addition, every year, literally hundreds of books on Chinese medicine are published, primarily in the People's Republic of China but also in Hong Kong and Taiwan. Further, there are approximately 30 TCM journals published in the PRC either monthly or bimonthly, each of which typically contains 20-30 articles on the latest TCM research, old doctors clinical experience, and the TCM treatment of Western disease categories.

This is all absolutely vital information for anyone trying to practice TCM here in the West. Textbooks are meant only for beginners. But Western practitioners, who all go into private practice, are typically asked to treat diseases which either did not get better on their own nor from the treatments of MDs, chiropractors, or osteopaths. Commonly, we are the last health care provider on a long list who the uncured patient sees as a last resort. Be that as it may, the overwhelming majority of Western practitioners of TCM have no personal access to the vast repository of Chinese medical literature *and never will* as long as they do not begin learning how to read Chinese. As a publisher, I can state categorically that this vast literature will never be translated into English for purely economic reasons. There are simply not enough English-speaking TCM practitioners worldwide to make such a venture financially profitable.

As I continued attempting to translate directly from Chinese medical sources, with each new Chinese medical term I learned and with each further sentence I could read, I found my understanding of TCM as a system increased exponentially. TCM as a system is largely based on the logic inherent in the Chinese language. That logic is not the same as that behind the structure of the English language. No matter how good the English language translator is, they can never fully express all the connotations nor the logic of presentation inherent in the original Chinese. This is a difficult thing to talk about. Those that already can read some TCM in Chinese will know what I am talking about. Those that do not will have a hard time really understanding how essential it is to read Chinese medicine in Chinese. Frequently, when I teach, I make the point that the reason I am the teacher and my audience are the students is because I can read some medical Chinese. Many of the students in my classes have been in practice just as long as I have. If I know anything about Chinese medicine which my peers do not know, it is only because I have access to information they do not. And that is information *in Chinese!*

For a number of years now, I have been stating in public that every student of TCM should learn to read simple, modern medical Chinese as part of their basic, entry level education. We would hardly accept a Western internist who only had access to a dozen, often inaccurately translated introductory texts. Yet the situation is exactly the same for practitioners of Traditional Chinese Medicine attempting to practice from the existing English language TCM literature. As I have mentioned above, I have demonstrated with two classes of students that undergraduates can begin translating *and publishing in juried professional venues* previously untranslated material within 3-4 months. Therefore, it is my belief that every Western school and college of TCM should teach *as a required course* a basic reading knowledge of modern medical Chinese. However, as of this writing, of the 50 American schools and colleges teaching acupuncture and Oriental medicine, only one teaches required courses in reading Chinese.

How can this be? First of all, most Westerners have the erroneous perception that Chinese is a very difficult language. It is not, at least not to read. Spoken Chinese with its tones may be difficult to pronounce and classical Chinese may be difficult to read, but modern medical Chinese as it appears in TCM texts and journal articles coming from the People's Republic of China is not. English is the difficult language; Chinese is not. English has tons of grammar; Chinese has comparatively very little. In addition, modern Chinese TCM is typically written in a very formulaic, repetitive style which makes it easy to read. Writers tend to use the same stock phrases over and over again, simply rearranging these in new ways to make fresh points. The one difficult thing about Chinese is that it is written by so-called characters and not by an alphabet. Really that is the only difficult thing about learning to read Chinese, and it is that problem, in large measure, this book attempts to solve for the beginner.

Secondly, most teachers who have attempted to teach Chinese at American acupuncture and Oriental medical colleges in the past have been native Chinese speakers. Typically, they approach the problem of teaching Chinese as if they were teaching college students enrolled in Chinese 101. Then they throw up their hands when acupuncture and TCM students find their classes too slow and irrelevant. Most Western acupuncture and Oriental medical students are adults who are going back to school to study for a change in career paths. Many of us are married and have other jobs. And almost every American school primarily holds its classes at night and on weekends. Therefore, our students are in a rush to get out of school. Every class they take needs to quickly reveal its relevance and show tangible results. Teaching Chinese medicine students Chinese as if they were going to read a newspaper or carry on a conversation is a waste of time for our students, and they quickly realize this.

However, if the teacher begins by showing their students the difference in technical meaning and implications between a single passage in Chinese and in an English language textbook, it is easy to demonstrate how important it is to get the right information. After all, we gather information about Chinese medicine which we intend to apply in a practical matter of great import, fiddling with other peoples' health. It is an easy matter to show how inaccurate and even downright erroneous much of the material in our currently existing English language textbooks is.

It is my experience that teachers at TCM schools and colleges should teach their students how to read medical Chinese by simply attempting to translate previously untranslated, clinically useful information right from the very first classes. There should be no lag time between introducing vocabulary and grammar and digging out the information necessary as a clinician. If the material the students attempt to read right from the first day of class is clinically useful information, they will immediately see the utility and importance of studying and attempting to read Chinese.

The third difficulty in teaching Western TCM students to read modern medical Chinese is the lack of textbooks. As mentioned above, the way one teaches Chinese to freshmen undergraduates in Chinese 101 is not the most pragmatic way to try to teach Chinese to beginning acupuncture and TCM students. As an extension of this, there simply have not been any textbooks designed specifically for teaching modern medical Chinese to this group of students. This book attempts to fill that need.

As a beginning Chinese textbook, this book is unlike any other of which I am aware. I have created it specifically to teach English speakers to read medical Chinese as quickly as possible. This book will not teach its readers how to carry on a conversation in Chinese nor to read a newspaper or even a Chinese menu. It is not organized like the typical Chinese language textbook. Mostly it is made up of lists which act as kinds of cheat sheets for novice translators to use who do not have the time nor inclination to study Chinese the way it is taught in academe. It may not be pretty, but it works, remembering that the prize is not a degree in Chinese but access to information as quickly as possible.

Western students always ask me how long it takes to learn Chinese. That is not the right question. The question should be, how long does it take to be able to read modern medical Chinese with the help of a dictionary and Chinese medical glossary. I do not *know* Chinese. I have not *learned* Chinese. I have only *studied* Chinese. It is probably only appropriate to say that a native speaker *knows* Chinese. I know more Chinese than I did last year, and doubtless I will know more Chinese next year than this. But one does not have to *know* Chinese in order to begin *translating* Chinese. And, in terms of this, it is never too late to begin trying to translate Chinese. Each sentence one translates is that much more Chinese medicine one will know and understand as it was originally conceived by the people who worked out this system and have proven its efficacy over no less than 2,500 years.

If a student learns to read medical Chinese during their initial training, they will be provided with the means to conduct their own research in the vaste and inexhaustible treasurehouse of the Chinese medical literature. Gaining access to this treasury allows one to continuously learn more and more about TCM. One is not limited to the facts one was able to memorize in school. One can continue their education indefinitely. In addition, they will be able to research difficult cases and study the clinical experiences of past great masters and life-long clinicians. Instead of reading a newspaper, novel, or magazine when the next patient blows off their appointment, one can translate an article in a Chinese TCM journal.

It is my experience that once one really begins to understand and appreciate what exists in the Chinese medical literature, one will wonder how they were ever able to practice without access to all this valuable information. Beside developing compassion and one's own healthy and healing qi, I can think of no more worthwhile study for the TCM practitioner than attempting to read medical Chinese. Several years ago, at Blue Poppy Press's invitation, a number of famous TCM practitioners and translators met to discuss translational issues and standards. Over the two day meeting, it became apparent that a hierarchy of authority arose spontaneously amongst the members of this group. When it came to matters pertaining to the understanding and practice of Chinese medicine, that hierarchy arranged itself according to how much Chinese one knew. (And I was nowhere near the head of the list.) Therefore, I can think of no more useful or important way for any Western student of TCM to spend their time than attempting to read Chinese medicine in Chinese. Hopefully, this book will make that study a little easier.

Bob Flaws
Boulder, CO

Table of Contents

1
Introduction

This workbook is designed to help you get started translating modern medical Chinese. It is intended for use primarily by Western acupuncture and Chinese medical students and practitioners. The outline and contents of this book are based on my "Learning to Read Modern Medical Chinese" seminars which I have been teaching in the United States for several years. This workbook can be used as part of a class with a real-life instructor or it can help you teach yourself to translate Chinese on your own at home. As I mention in the Preface, it is a "down and dirty" approach to learning to read Chinese created by someone who has taught himself and who wishes to share a few tricks with other like-minded individuals. There are many other books available in the market to help you learn Chinese. A list of some of these is included in the annotated bibliography at the back of this book.

Rather than progressing through a series of grammar and vocabulary exercises like most foreign language textbooks do, we will learn to read modern medical Chinese mainly by trying to read it with the aid of Chinese-English dictionaries, Chinese medical dictionaries, "cheat sheets", and glossaries. We will begin with a brief introduction to the Chinese language. Then we will learn how to look up words in a Chinese-English dictionary. *This is the single most important skill necessary to learn how to read modern medical Chinese.* From there, we will go directly to a series of exercises practicing translation. The more interested you are in this endeavor, the more books you will want to read on the Chinese language. And the more you learn about the Chinese language, the easier this endeavor will be. However, besides a certain amount of verbal intuition, the main quality necessary to successfully translate modern medical Chinese is *dogged perserverance.*

This book will not help you learn to *speak* Chinese. In it, I pay no attention to pronunciation. Chinese is a very difficult language to learn to pronounce correctly. One of the things that make speaking Chinese difficult is that it is a tonal language. In standard Mandarin, there are five tones. In Shanghainese and Cantonese, there are more like 10. Even Chinese cannot speak together unless they speak *pu tong hua* or standard speech, and even then you see them writing characters on their palms trying to make themselves understood.

Although speaking Chinese is a wonderful skill, I do not believe it is a necessary skill for translating the Chinese medical literature. There is a big difference between being able to read a language and being able to speak a language. My main concern is to help you gain firsthand access to the Chinese medical literature. To do that, it is reading comprehension which is the key. Certainly, if you go to study in China, the more Chinese you speak, the more you will get out of your stay. But for the average Western student or practitioner living in the West, the most important thing is to learn how to read modern medical Chinese.

2
About the Chinese Language

The Chinese language is part of the Sino-Tibetan language group. What this mainly means to us is that, in structure, logic, and vocabulary, Chinese is radically unlike any Indo-European language. Unlike French, Spanish, German, or even Hebrew and Russian, it is *totally foreign*. Written Chinese, unlike all the above, is not an alphabet-based language. Rather it is written with characters or ideograms (also called logograms by some sinologists). Each ideogram stands for a word.[1] These ideograms were derived from pictograms or pictures of the concepts they represented. Therefore, one could say that Chinese uses a symbol-based system of writing. This also means that each character must be memorized as a unit. One cannot sound out a word as one does in English and, when one has sounded it out, then understand what word it is. In fact, it is possible in Chinese to know the meaning of a character without knowing how the character is pronounced.[2]

In terms of dealing with characters as opposed to phonemes, Chinese is a hard language to learn to read even for Chinese. To use today's jargon, there is a very steep initial learning curve. The good news is that, after one masters the initial hurdle of dealing with characters instead of an alphabet, the grammar is easier than, say, Latin, German, or Sanskrit. Words have no gender and there is no declension of nouns. There is not even any number (*i.e.*, singular or plural). There are no inflections (those pesky word ending changes common in most Indo-European languages), and no conjugation of verbs. In fact, there is no past, present, or future.[3]

Here are several very easy Chinese characters. I bet you can remember them even by only looking at them once. They are a good example of the fact that this character-based system of writing is not all that hard and is certainly not impossible.

一	One
二	Two
三	Three
人	Human being, person
口	Mouth
十	Ten
天	Heaven
木	Tree or wood

---

[1] "Here much of the disagreement centers on a controversial question: What constitutes a word? For some, a word in Chinese is a syllable in speech and a character in writing. For others, syllable and character represent at most not a word but rather a morpheme, the smallest unit of meaning. By this definition, a word may in fact include more than one syllablel and be represented by more than one character." John De Francis, *The Chinese Language: Fact and Fantasy*, Univeristy of Hawaii Press, Honolulu, 1984, p. 72

[2] That Chinese is a symbol-based system of writing is a bit of an oversimplification. In fact, 90% of Chinese characters do include some phonetic marker.

[3] "Chinese grammar is probably easier than French grammar with its complex verb conjugations, agreement of nouns and adjectives, and other features that are largely lacking in Chinese." De Francis, *ibid.*, p. 52

Complicated & simplified characters

Because the recognition and memorization of characters presents an initially difficult challenge, the percentage of literate Chinese has, until recently, always been quite low. Rather than a hereditary nobility based on military prowess, the Chinese evolved a meritocracy based on ability to read Chinese. This meritocracy of the literate was a direct outgrowth of the difficulties inherent in reading Chinese.

One of the main goals of the Chinese Communist Party when it took over power in 1949 was to increase education so as to modernize the country and upgrade its peoples' standard of living. A necessary first step in this modernization was to increase the literacy rates in China. Recognizing the difficulties inherent in learning to read the Chinese character-based language, the regime in the People's Republic of China instituted a language reform in 1956.

For hundreds of years or more, Chinese scholars have used a simplified version of the characters with fewer strokes when writing for everyday purposes. When composing something for publication or propagation, they would use the more complicated, "official" versions instead. These more complicated versions have more strokes than the everyday way of writing. The Chinese Communists adopted these simplified, "everyday" characters as the new official standard within the PRC. They then also created a number of new, simplified versions of old, complicated characters. Therefore, many of these simplified characters are not a new invention. They have been in use for hundreds, if not thousands, of years. Below, as an example, is the character for medicine, *yi*, written first on the left in the complicated form and then secondly on the right in its simplified form.

醫 医

As you can see, there's a lot less strokes to remember in the simplified character than in the old, "official", more complicated version. Here are some other examples of simplified versus complicated or traditional characters.

貝	贝	shell
門	门	door
藥	药	herbs, medicinals
馬	马	horse
順	顺	compliant, favorable, normally flowing¡

It is true that, in "greater China", *i.e.*, including Hong Kong, Taiwan, and Singapore as well as in overseas Chinese communities around the world, there is an on-going debate about these so-called simplified characters. Traditionalists say this reduction in strokes over-simplifies the characters and loses meaning in the process. For instance, in the character *yi* for medicine, the complicated form contains the bottle radical (酉) on the bottom. This implies medicine stored in a bottle. On the top, we have an arrow in a container on the left (医), while, on the right, there's a hand making a jerky movement symbolizing someone taking this arrow out of its container (殳).

(Agreed, this "hand" is pretty stylized!) Thus the complicated character for medicine tells us that, at the time this character was created, medicine in China was a combination of administering medicinals stored in bottles and piercing patients with arrows (probably initially to drive out evil spirits).[4] Be that as it may, the simplification of writing carried out in the PRC since 1949 has made Chinese much easier to read for beginners. Read: you and me. In fact, those simplified characters that have always been used as a sort of shorthand by Chinese can be found in Hong Kong, Taiwan, and overseas Chinese communities. It is only the Communist-created ones that are found only in the PRC.

This book only really deals with reading the simplified characters used in the PRC. We will talk briefly about what to do when you come across complicated characters. However, I highly recommend that you begin the same way that modern Chinese children in the PRC begin—with the simplified characters. This means that, for now, your reading will be confined to books and articles published in the People's Republic of China. Books and articles published in Hong Kong, Taiwan, Singapore, and in overseas Chinese communities around the world typically use the complicated characters.[5]

Then you may ask, won't this limit my reading? Yes, theoretically, it will. However, there is so much available on all aspects of Chinese medicine printed in the People's Republic of China in simplified characters that you could translate your entire life without ever exhausting what is available in simplified characters. Even all the great Chinese medical classics have been printed using simplified characters. The People's Republic of China outpublishes all other Chinese sources of information on Chinese medicine. So, in reality, this simplification of characters is a blessing for *wai* (外, outside) *guo* (国, country) *ren* (人, people), *i.e.*, foreigners, such as ourselves.

Mandarin & Pu Tong Hua

If someone says they *speak* Chinese, it is appropriate to ask whether they speak Mandarin or some other regional dialect.[6] The word Mandarin comes from the Portuguese which in turn comes from the Latin, *mandare*, to order. Mandarins are what early Europeans called the Confucian scholars who were the officials of the Chinese imperial bureacracy. Therefore, their language was also called Mandarin. However, Mandarin is nothing other than the regional dialect spoken in the capital, *Beijing*. We can say then that Mandarin is really nothing other than *bei* (北, northern) *jing* (京, capital) *hua* (话, speech).

---

[4] This explanation of the derivation of the complex way of writing the character *yi* or medicine is from Ping-gam Go's *Understanding Chinese Characters by Their Ancestral Forms*, third edition, Simplex Publications, SF, CA, 1995, p. 32

[5] William McNaughton, in *Reading & Writing Chinese*, Charles E. Tuttle Co., Rutland, VT, 1996, on page 17-18 says: "To learn only these short forms, however, is a great mistake. In so doing students effectively cut themselves off from all the traditional Chinese literary and historical material as well as from most of the Chinese books available in Western libraries, which were written (and printed) before the process of simplification began. Students who can read only the short form will be able to read what Mao Tse-tung wrote, but they will be unable to read what Mao Tse-tung himself read..." Although that is an interesting point, most materials currently available about the clinical practice of Chinese medicine *are* printed in simplified characters. In addition, all the great premodern Chinese medical classics have also been issued in simplified character versions. So one is not necessarily limited to only modern sources.

[6] Actually, so-called regional dialects are much more than dialects. In fact, they might be called separate languages, since speakers of Shanghainese, Hakka, or Cantonese cannot understand each other or speakers of mandarin.

In 1949, in an effort to turn an empire into a united and cohesive country, the Chinese Communists adopted Mandarin or *Bei Jing hua* as the standard dialect of China for the whole country. However, they renamed it *pu* (普, universal, common) *tong* (通, communicate) *hua* (话, speech). This means that virtually all Chinese under 45 years of age speak *pu tong hua* as well as their regional dialect. Of course, there are regional accents when speaking *pu tong hua* and some people have learned this "foreign" language better than others. Nevertheless, the adoption of *pu tong hua* has created a single national language spoken from Heilongjiang (黑龙江 , black dragon river) in the northeast to Urumuqi in the northwest and from Hainan in the south to Beijing in the north.

Be that as it may, all Chinese (at least all Han people) have always written Chinese the same no matter how they spoke their regional dialect. An old person from Suzhou may not be able to speak to another old person from Guizhou, but they can read each others letters. This means that we don't have to worry about whether something is written in Mandarin or Cantonese. All *written* Chinese is the same!

Pinyin

During the 1950s, recognizing the problems their system of writing presents in the modern world, the Chinese flirted with the idea of scrapping their character-based way of writing and adopting the Roman alphabet. At that time, it was the Russians who were the Chinese Communists best friends. Professionals who went to school in 50's all studied Russian. So when the Chinese tried to phoneticize the writing of their language with the Roman alphabet in the 1950s, they did so based on a Russian's attempts to pronounce Chinese. A Russian knows to pronounce zh as j and q as ch. This is why an English speaker trying to pronounce Chinese from its Pinyin spelling rarely even comes close to the Chinese.

In addition, Chinese is a tonal language. The same syllable pronounced in a different tone has a different meaning. For instance, *ma* when pronounced in the first tone means mother but pronounced in the second tone means hemp, in the third tone means horse, and in the fourth tone means to curse or swear. In other words, just the Roman letters *m* and *a* written together can mean a number of different words depending on their pronounciation. To make matters even worse, there are five different Chinese words spelled *ma* and pronounced in the first tone, four different second tone *ma* words, six different third tone *ma* words, and two different fourth tone *ma* words, not to mention two more *ma* words spoken without tone. All are written with different Chinese characters. Therefore, it is easy to see that simply writing the Pinyin *ma,* there is no way to differentiate which *ma* is actually meant.

Below we will talk about other ways of romanizing the *pu tong hua* or Mandarin pronunciation of Chinese characters. However, within the Western profession of acupuncture and Chinese medicine, Pinyin has been adopted as the *de facto* standard (even though no English speaker can actually pronounce it correctly on first sight!). Therefore, I will use Pinyin from here on out whenever I romanize anything in this workbook, such as acupuncture points or Chinese medicinal names. Nevertheless, because Chinese is a character-based language, you can learn to read a word and know its English language meaning without ever knowing how it is pronounced in China (whether in *pu tong hua,* Cantonese, Shanghainese, Fujianese, etc.).

3
The Development of Chinese Writing

Chinese characters are the oldest, continually used form of writing in the world. Although there is evidence of character-based writing in what is now China in the Stone Age, the written historical record of the Chinese language begins in the Shang dynasty (16th-11th centuries BCE). During this time, shamans used a method of divination based on heating the undershells of turtles and the shoulder bones of oxen in a fire. The cracks which were produced were then "read" similar to a Roman augur's reading of chicken entrails or shooting stars. In order to keep track of these predictions, the shamans created a pictographic system of writing which they carved alongside the divinatory cracks. These characters are called oracle bone characters, and about one third of all oracle bone characters currently archived have been deciphered.

Because these early pictographs or ideograms were carved with a sharp blade into a hard surface, they tended to be highly stylized. After writing on tortoise plastrums and ox shoulder blades, early Chinese went on to write by carving on stone and metal. In older times, there was no "official" standard way to write a word, and the same word would often have a number of variant writings. As time went on, however, the shapes of the characters became more uniform. Prior to the unification of China in the third century BCE by Shi Huang Di, the most common form of writing was called large seal script or *da quan*. From this, Shi Huang Di had created what is now called small seal script or *xiao quan*. This became the standard of official writing throughout the empire.

In the Han dynasty (206 BCE to 220 CE), clerical script or *li shu* developed. This was a simpler form of writing used at first only for unofficial business. Towards the end of the Han dynasty, *kai shu* or regular script was developed. This is the form of Chinese writing which is the model used for printed characters in books and newspapers and is the style learned by Chinese school children similar to how Western children begin with "block printing." This style is very legible, regular, and distinct.

Below is a chart showing the evolution in writing several common characters from ancient Shang dynasty forms to modern styles of writing. As you can see, the shapes of the characters generally go from naturalistic to highly stylized, and the style of the lines themselves are dependent upon the media with which the characters are written.

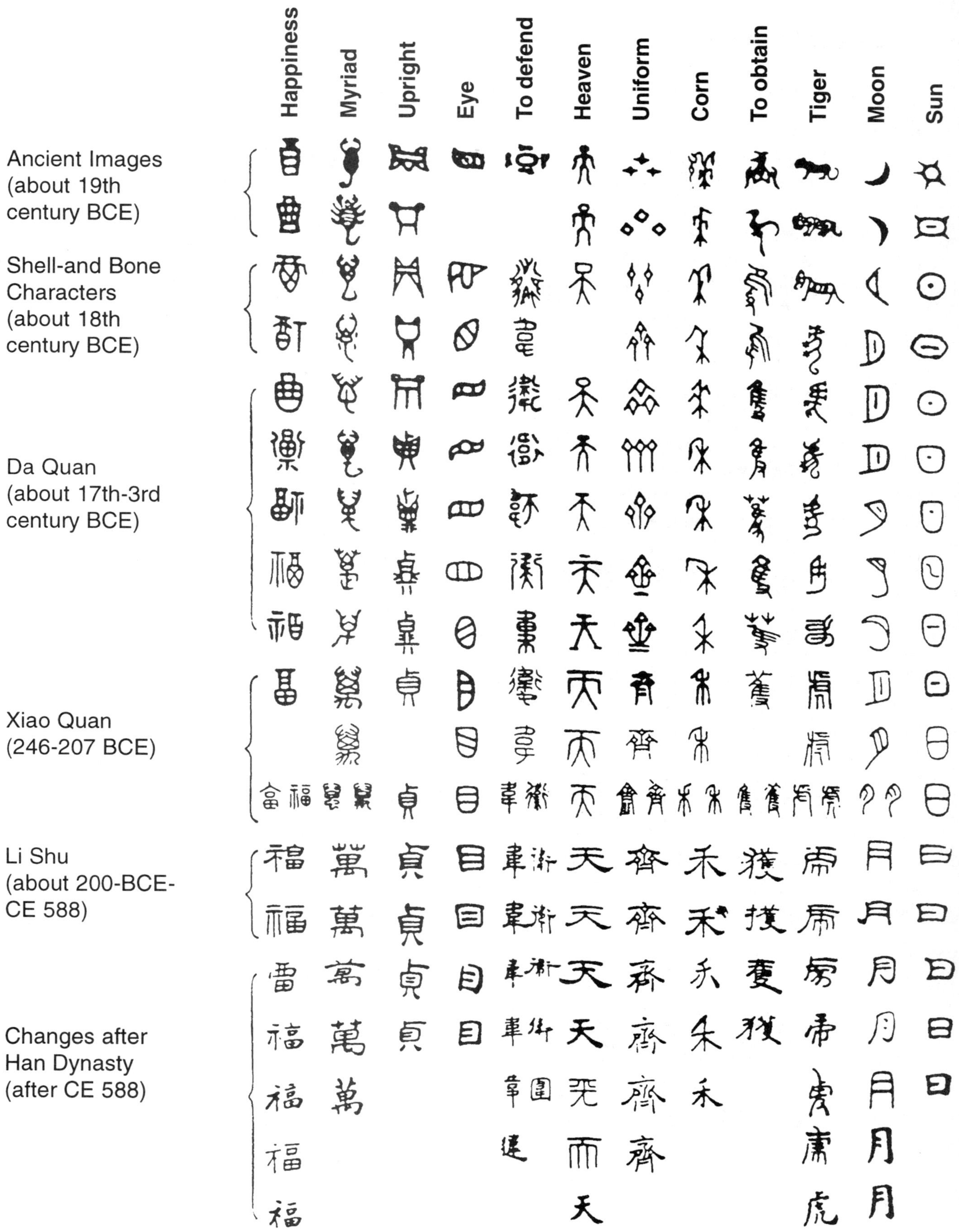
Happiness
Myriad
Upright
Eye
To defend
Heaven
Uniform
Corn
To obtain
Tiger
Moon
Sun
Ancient Images (about 19th century BCE)
Shell-and Bone Characters (about 18th century BCE)
Da Quan (about 17th-3rd century BCE)
Xiao Quan (246-207 BCE)
Li Shu (about 200-BCE-CE 588)
Changes after Han Dynasty (after CE 588)

Six Different Styles of Chinese Writing.
(Reproduced from Williams's *Middle Kingdom*.)

When written by hand with a brush pen, there are two other styles of writing Chinese characters. These are called *xing shu* or running, moving script and *cao shu* or grass script. Both of these are "cursive" forms of handwriting. *Xing shu* is more regular and easier to read, while *cao shu* is so cursive, fluid, and simplified to the point of abstraction that it is almost impossible to read unless you are used to that person's handwriting *and* know what the subject is about! We will not be trying to read either seal styles or running and grass styles. Everything about Chinese medicine which we will attempt to read as beginners is printed in some form of *kai shu* or regular script.

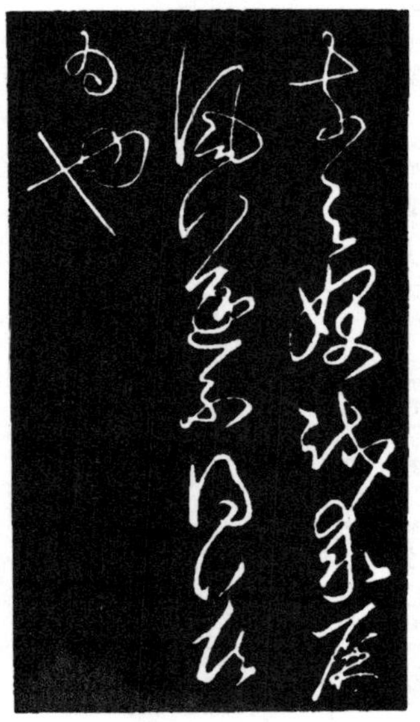

Cao shu by Wang Xi-zhi

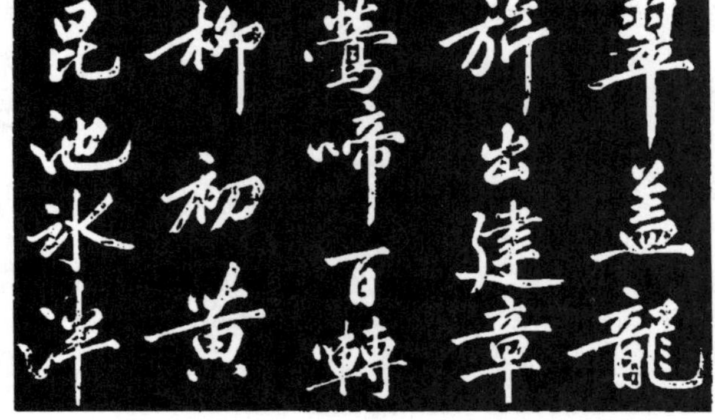

Xing shu by Huang Ting-jian

In addition to these major styles of Chinese writing, there are innumerable personal variations. Two such personal variations are shown below.

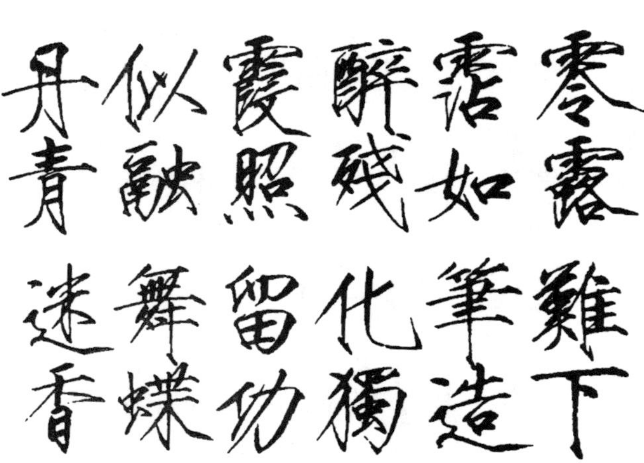

Xing shu by the Song emperor Hui Zong

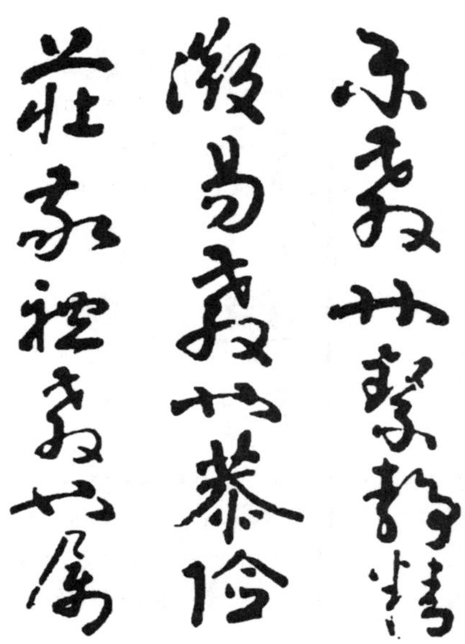

Anonymous *xing shu*

Six ways Chinese characters were/are created

Basically, each character is a picture. However, each picture stands for a word, and some words are abstract concepts which are difficult to pictorialize. Therefore, we can identify six basic ways Chinese characters were or are created. These six basic types of characters are:

1. Pictographs
2. Symbols, *i.e.*, characters depicting abstract concepts
3. Sound-meaning compounds, *i.e.*, characters formed from a phonetic and a radical
4. Sound loans, *i.e.*, characters borrowed without adding a radical
5. Meaning-meaning compounds
6. Reclarified compounds[1]

Pictographs are pictures of the physical objects which they symbolize. For instance, 日 (*ri*) stands for sun. This is not so easy to see when written in *kai shu*, but, if we go back to its Shang dynasty form ⊙, it is easy to see. Likewise, 月 (*yue*) stands for moon. Its Shang dynasty form was written 𝄐 .

Characters depicting abstract concepts are a little harder to pictorialize. The characters for up and down or above and below, 上 and 下, are basically symbols. Meaning-meaning compounds are likewise simply more complex symbols where two or more characters are put together. Basically, these meaning-meaning compound characters tell a story. Take, for instance, the character for the word "good" (好, *hao*). It is composed of two parts. On the left there is a woman (女) and on the right there is a child (子). According to the ancient Chinese way of seeing things, a woman with a child is a "good" thing.

Characters formed from a phonetic and a radical also symbolize something which is otherwise difficult to pictorialize. When the need arose for a character whose meaning was difficult to illustrate with simple pictures, the character was often created by borrowing an existing character whose spoken form had the same pronunciation as the wanted word. In this case, a meaning marker or radical was added to the character for the well-known homonym. This then created a new character based in a combination of sound and sense. Take for example the character for grass or herb, *cao*. It has two parts. The radical at the top (艹) shows grass growing, while the bottom part is the character for the word "early" (早, *zao*). The word "early" is pronounced *zao* and the word for "grass" is pronounced *cao*. These were close enough that, with the addition of the grass radical, one gets the character 草. This type of character is called a sound-meaning compound.

Sometimes when a new character is needed, an old, possibly obsolete one is borrowed without adding a radical. In this case, the old character is simply invested with a new meaning. For instance, the character *lai* (来) which means to come originally depicted a kind of wheat. However, because the name of this kind of wheat was pronounced the same as the word "to

---

[1] Some Chinese language scholars only recognize four types of characters. In that case, the four types are the first four in this list.

come", the character was adopted for that purpose without making any changes or additions to it. This is called a sound loan character.

Reclarified compounds are a little more difficult to describe. Over time, languages change. Perhaps a character came to mean a number of different things and there now was confusion over exactly what was meant when this character was used. Did it mean this or did it mean that. Originally, the character 廷 (*ting*) meant "court". However, this could mean anyone's court or the king's court. In order to clarify whose court people were talking about (actually, writing about), a new character was created to clarify this issue. Thus the character 庭 came to mean specifically the "king's court" as opposed to your and my court. This is what is meant by a reclarified compound.

Happily, when it comes to translating modern medical Chinese, one does not really need to know where a character came from or how it developed. As long as we are reading modern medical Chinese, what we are most concerned with is the character's current medical definition and usage, and these we can get by looking the word up in our Chinese-English dictionary.

4
Counting Strokes

Most Chinese-English dictionaries are arranged alphabetically by Pinyin romanization. However, if you do not already know the pronunciation of the Chinese word and its Pinyin romanization, you cannot use this alphabetical system. Since Chinese characters are not alphabet-based, this makes looking Chinese words up in a dictionary more difficult than in English. There are two skills which must be mastered before one can look up a word in an Chinese-English dictionary.

The first is counting strokes. Characters in Chinese character indexes are typically arranged by counting the number of strokes. Since different characters have different numbers of strokes, it is possible to list all characters with six strokes, those with seven, or those with any other number of strokes. However, before one can count strokes, one must first know what are the strokes in written Chinese. Although counting strokes may, at first, seem extremely easy and self-evident, because the Chinese write certain strokes in certain ways if one is not familiar with the repertoire of strokes, one may easily miscount.

In written Chinese, there are six basic or simple strokes:

Strokes	Names	Examples
`	dot	不
一	horizontal stroke	不
丨	vertical stroke	不
丿	left-falling stroke	八
＼	right-falling stroke	八
✓	rising stroke	汉

Then there are another 17 strokes which are complicated stokes. These contain hooks or turns or are made by combining two or more of the above basic strokes.

Strokes	Names	Examples
⼀	horizontal + hook stroke	你
亅	vertical + hook stroke	小
⺄	slanting + hook stroke	我

⌊	vertical + rising stroke
⼽	horizontal + turned back stroke
⌐	vertical + turned back stroke
⼃	left-falling + dot
⼃	left-falling + turned back stroke
⼅	horizontal + left-falling stroke
⌐	vertical + bend stroke
⼅	horizontal + turned back + hook stroke
⼅	vertical + bend + hook stroke
⌐	horizontal + turned back + vertical stroke
⌐	vertical + turned back + turned back + hook stroke
⌐	horizontal + turned back + bend + left-falling stroke
⼄	horizontal + turned back + bend + hook stroke
⼄	horizontal + turned back + bend + hook stroke

Once one knows the basic strokes used in writing Chinese, one must also learn the basic order in writing these strokes.

Stroke Order Rules

1. From top to bottom
This means that strokes forming the upper part of a character should be written before those forming the lower part. For instance:

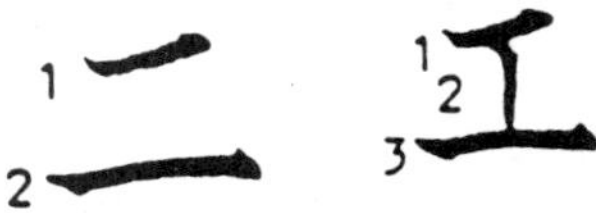

2. From left to right
This means that the writing of a left-falling stroke or stroke on the left side should precede the writing of a right-falling stroke or stroke on the right side. For instance:

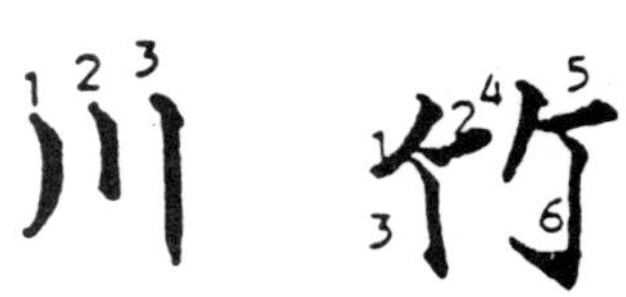

3. From outer to inner

This means strokes on the outside of a character should be written before strokes on the inside. For instance:

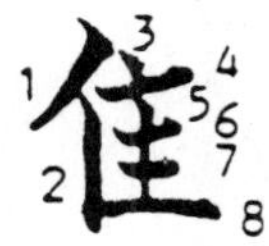

4. Seal last

This means that sealing strokes should be last to be written. For instance:

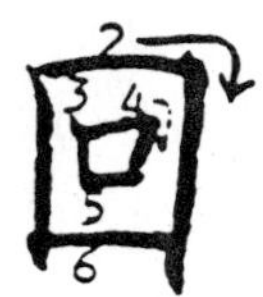

5. From horizontal to vertical

This means that the writing of horizontal strokes should precede the writing of vertical strokes. For instance:

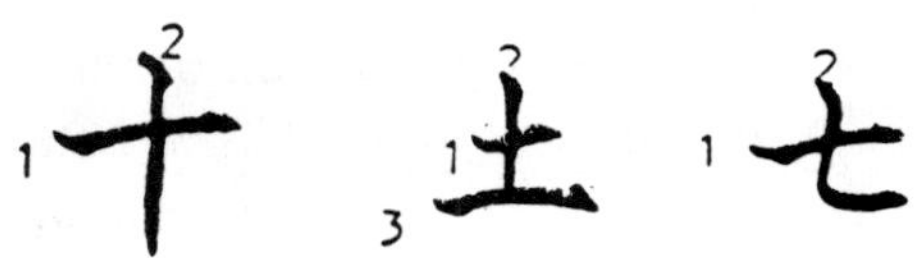

6. Middle first

This means that middle strokes should be written before strokes on both sides. For instance:

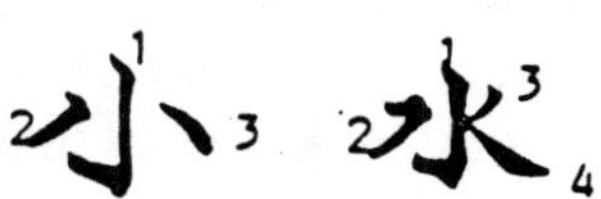

Below are some sample characters with the number of their strokes counted in succession according to Chinese rules for stroke order.

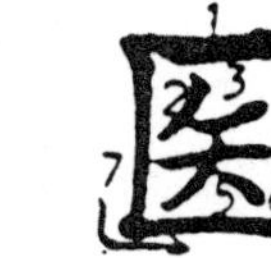

Exercise: Cover the answer column on the right with a piece of paper. Then count the number of strokes in each of the following characters on the left and write this in the parentheses to the side of each character. When you are done, remove the piece of paper covering the answers and see how you have done.

Characters   **Answers**

1. 阴   (   )   yin (6)
2. 阳   (   )   yang (6)
3. 木   (   )   wood (4)
4. 面   (   )   face (9)
5. 土   (   )   earth (3)

6. 金　　　(　)　　　　metal (8)
7. 水　　　(　)　　　　water (4)
8. 药　　　(　)　　　　medicinals (9)
9. 治　　　(　)　　　　treatment (8)
10. 泻　　　(　)　　　drain (8)
11. 经　　　(　)　　　channels (8)
12. 络　　　(　)　　　network vessels (9)
13. 针　　　(　)　　　needle or acupuncture (7)
14. 灸　　　(　)　　　moxibustion (7)
15. 克　　　(　)　　　grams (7)
16. 汤　　　(　)　　　decoction (6)
17. 病　　　(　)　　　disease (10)
18. 表　　　(　)　　　exterior (8)
19. 痢　　　(　)　　　dysentery (12)
20. 伤　　　(　)　　　damage (6)

Although we all say we are busy people, there are times in each of our days when we have nothing to do. So we flip through a magazine or turn on the TV. When I was a student in China in 1983, there was very little to do in the evenings. So I purchased a children's primer on how to write Chinese and practiced writing Chinese characters. When I finally decided to try to read Chinese in earnest (notice I did not say try to *learn* Chinese in earnest), my practice of writing Chinese characters with their proper strokes paid off. Therefore, below are some character writing practice sheets. I recommend photocopying them so that you can do them over and over. The more you are used to writing the basic Chinese character strokes, the easier it will be to count strokes in the characters you are trying to look up and to retain the shapes of characters in your mind's eye.

Trace each of the following strokes in the direction indicated:

ノ (↙)	ノ	ノ	ノ	ノ	ノ	ノ	ノ	ノ
＼ (↘)	＼	＼	＼	＼	＼	＼	＼	＼
一 (→)	一	一	一	一	一	一	一	一
｜ (↓)	｜	｜	｜	｜	｜	｜	｜	｜
ヽ (↘)	ヽ	ヽ	ヽ	ヽ	ヽ	ヽ	ヽ	ヽ
㇕ (㇕)	㇕	㇕	㇕	㇕	㇕	㇕	㇕	㇕

Now copy each stroke in the squares of each row:

Trace each character in the correct stroke order:

Copy each character in the correct stroke order, using crossed boxes to postition each one correctly:

八	bā
不	bù
大	dà
一	yī
五	wǔ

Trace the following characters:

身	身	身	身	身	身	身	身	身	身
体	体	体	体	体	体	体	体	体	体
六	六	六	六	六	六	六	六	六	六
七	七	七	七	七	七	七	七	七	七
九	九	九	九	九	九	九	九	九	九
小	小	小	小	小	小	小	小	小	小
他	他	他	他	他	他	他	他	他	他

Copy the following characters:

身									shēn
体									tǐ
六									liù
七									qī
九									jiǔ
小									xiǎo
他									tā

5
Identifying radicals

Identifying radicals is the second basic skill in looking a character up in a Chinese-English dictionary. However, before we go any further, we must first make sure you own a Chinese-English dictionary. Because we are going to be reading books and articles from the People's Republic of China, I highly recommend that you purchase a Chinese-English dictionary based on those prepared by the Foreign Language Institute in Beijing using the simplified characters and Pinyin. Please see the bibliography in the back for more information about Chinese-English dictionaries.

Assuming that we all have a Chinese-English dictionary in hand, the vast majority of Chinese characters include a section which is called the radical. The radical is the key for looking up the character in the dictionary. Although Chinese characters are not made up of letters as in an alphabet, they are made up of building blocks. Modern Chinese-English dictionaries published in the People's Republic of China all have a "Radical Index" in the front of the book.

The Radical Index from *the Pinyin Chinese-English Dictionary,* published jointly by the Commercial Press, Beijing & Hong Kong, and John Wiley and sons, Inc. New York, 1991, is shown below. Starting up at the left hand corner of the chart we see the character 画. This means "stroke". 一 means "one" and 画 means "stroke". (Literally, this second character means "painting".) Under this heading, there are then seven radicals numbered with Arabic numerals on the far left. These are all the radicals which are written with a single stroke of the pen. As you will see, number seven has two alternate forms.

Below radical number seven, there are the Chinese characters 二 画. These mean "two strokes". 二 means "two". Under this heading there are 31 more radicals. Radicals number eight through 39 are all written with two strokes. A couple of these also have two alternate forms. Radicals 33 and 34 seem to be exactly the same radicals. They are. However, when that radical appears on the left side of the character it is radical 33, and when it appears on the right side of the character it is number 34. The characters in parentheses next to radical 33 say *zai zuo,* 在左. *Zai* means "location" or "located", and *zuo* means "left". That means that the two characters in parentheses next to radical number 34 must mean "located on the right." How do I know this? The character *zai* is the same in both cases. If *zuo* means "left", it only stands to reason that the other character (右) means "right". It does; it is *you.*

Following down this list of radicals, after radical 39, there are the two characters, 三画 . By now you should know what they mean even without looking them up or being told. See if you can figure them out. You've seen the right character two previous times in this chapter so far. Yup, you're right. 三 means three. So that means you also should be able to figure out the Chinese numbers for four through 14. If you find the radicals written with fourteen strokes (十 [10] + 四 [4] = 十四[14]), you will see there is only one, number 226. But then you have another category numbered 227 but headed by only a line. The two Chinese characters here say *yu lei,*

部　首　检　字
Radical　Index

（一）　部首目录

部首左边的号码表示部首的次序

一　画		35	又	70	ヨ（彑彐）	105	中	140	业	175	缶	209	鱼
1	、	36	乚	71	弓	106	贝	141	目	176	耒	九　画	
2	一	37	厶	72	己（巳）	107	见	142	田	177	舌	210	音
3	丨	38	凵	73	女	108	父	143	由	178	竹（⺮）	211	革
4	丿	39	匕	74	子（孑）	109	气	144	申	179	臼	212	是
5	乛	三　画		75	马	110	牛（牜）	145	罒	180	自	213	骨
6	乛	40	氵	76	幺	111	手	146	皿	181	血	214	香
7	乙（乁乚）	41	忄	77	纟（糸）	112	毛	147	钅	182	舟	215	鬼
二　画		42	丬（爿）	78	巛	113	攵	148	矢	183	羽	216	食
8	冫	43	亡	79	小（⺍）	114	片	149	禾	184	艮（⻀）	十　画	
9	亠	44	广	四　画		115	斤	150	白	七　画		217	高
10	讠	45	丷	80	灬	116	爪（爫）	151	瓜	185	言	218	鬲
11	二	46	门	81	心	117	尺	152	鸟	186	辛	219	髟
12	十	47	辶	82	斗	118	月	153	皮	187	辰	十一　画	
13	厂	48	工	83	火	119	殳	154	癶	188	麦	220	麻
14	ナ	49	土（士）	84	文	120	欠	155	矛	189	走	221	鹿
15	匚	50	艹	85	方	121	风	156	疋	190	赤	十二　画	
16	卜（⼘）	51	廾	86	户	122	氏	六　画		191	豆	222	黑
17	刂	52	大	87	礻	123	比	157	羊（⺶⺷）	192	束	十三　画	
18	冖	53	尢	88	王	124	毋	158	关	193	酉	223	鼓
19	冂	54	寸	89	主	125	水	159	米	194	豕	224	鼠
20	宀	55	扌	90	天（夭）	五　画		160	齐	195	里	十四　画	
21	亻	55	弋	91	韦	126	立	161	衣	196	足	225	鼻
22	厂	57	巾	92	耂	127	疒	162	亦（亦）	197	采	—	
23	人（入）	58	口	93	廿（卅）	128	穴	163	耳	198	豸	226	余类
24	八（丷）	59	囗	94	木	129	衤	164	臣	199	谷		
25	乂	60	山	95	不	130	夬	165	聿	200	身		
26	勹	61	屮	96	犬	131	玉	166	西（覀）	201	角		
27	刀（⼑）	62	彳	97	歹	132	示	167	束	八　画			
28	力	63	彡	98	瓦	133	去	168	亚	202	青		
29	儿	64	夕	99	牙	134	此	169	而	203	其		
30	几（⼏）	65	夂	100	车	135	甘	170	页	204	雨		
31	マ	66	丸	101	戈	136	石	171	至	205	非		
32	卩	67	尸	102	止	137	龙	172	光	206	齿		
33	阝（在左）	68	饣	103	日	138	戊	173	虍	207	隹		
34	阝（在右）	69	犭	104	曰	139	⺌	174	虫	208	金		

"remaining kinds or types". This is a group of 12 characters which have no radicals. We'll come back to these in a bit.

What are radicals?

Radicals are almost all Chinese words in their own right. They are 226 seminal or key words or strokes which are used as building blocks to create more complex characters. Each radical not only has a number in the Radical Index but a name or meaning to native Chinese-speakers. The meanings of the 226 radicals are given below. When learning Chinese at a university, your teacher will typically require that you memorize the meanings of each of these radicals. I never have. Many of them you will learn as you go along. It doesn't hurt to memorize them, but you do not need to do so to proceed. Note, in a few instances, I have not been able to identify the original meaning conveyed by a radical. Therefore, some spaces for the names or meanings of the radicals are blank after their number.

One stroke radicals
1. Dot
2. Horizontal line or one
3. Vertical line or down
4. Left-slanting line
5. Horizontal + hook
6. Horizontal + break
7. Vertical + bend + hook

Two stroke radicals
8. Ice
9. Lid
10. Words
11. Two
12. Ten
13. Cliff
14. Grasping hand
15. Box or within
16. Foretell
17. Knife
18. Cover or crown
19. Borders
20. Left one
21. Human
22. Partial
23. Human
24. Eight
25.
26. Wrap
27. Knife

28. Strength
29. Legs
30. Table
31.
32. Seal
33. Mound (or small village)
34. Mound (or big village)
35. Also
36. Long stride
37. Go
38. Can
39. Spoon

Three stroke radicals
40. Water
41. Heart
42. Bed
43. Conquer
44. Shelter
45. Roof
46. Door
47. Road
48. Work
49. Earth (soldier)
50. Grass
51. Play
52. Big
53. Lame
54. Inch
55. Hand

56. Shoot
57. Napkin
58. Mouth
59. Fence
60. Mountain
61. Sprout
62. Double man
63. Shape
64. Evening
65. Summer
66. Pill
67. Foot
68. Food or to eat
69. Dog
70. Broom
71. Bow
72. Oneself (cease)
73. Woman
74. Son
75. Horse
76. Number one
77. Silk
78. Stream
79. Small

Four stroke radicals
80. Fire
81. Heart
82. Measure
83. Fire
84. Support
85. Direction
86. Family
87. Show
88. King
89.
90. Heaven
91. Leather
92. Old
93. Twenty
94. Tree
95. No
96. Dog
97. Bad
98. Tile

99. Tooth
100. Chariot
101. Spear
102. Stop
103. Sun
104. Say
105. Center
106. Cowry
107. See
108. Father
109. Qi
110. Cow
111. Hand
112. Hair
113. Tap
114. Slice
115. Ax
116. Claw
117. Cubit
118. Moon (or meat)
119. Strike
120. Lacking
121. Wind
122. Clan
123. Compare
124. Learn
125. Water

Five stroke radicals
126. Stand
127. Disease
128. Cave
129. Clothes
130.
131. Jade
132. Show
133. Leave
134.
135. Sweet
136. Stone
137. Dragon
138. Fifth stem
139. Knowledge received from above
140. Property
141. Eye

142. Field
143. Entrance
144. Express
145. Net
146. Vessel
147. Gold or metal
148. Arrow
149. Rice stalk
150. White
151. Melon
152. Bird
153. Skin
154. Climb
155. Lance
156.

Six stroke radicals
157. Sheep
158.
159. Rice
160. Uniform, neat
161. Robes
162. Even
163. Ear
164. Officer
165.
166. West
167. Wheat
168. Second
169. And
170. Page
171. Reach
172. Light
173. Tiger
174. Insect
175. Pottery
176. Plough
177. Tongue
178. Bamboo
179. Uncle
180. From
181. Blood
182. Ship
183. Feather

184. Good

Seven stroke radicals
185. Speech
186. Difficult
187. Time
188. Wheat
189. Run
190. Red
191. Bean
192. Sheaf
193. Chief
194. Pig
195. Li (unit of measurement)
196. Leg
197. Pick
198. Leopard
199. Valley
200. Body
201. Horn

Eight stroke radicals
202. Green
203.
204. Rain
205. Not
206. Front tooth
207. Turtle
208. Single
209. Gold
210. Fish

Nine stroke radicals
211. Sound
212. Revolution
213. Correct
214. Bone
215. Aroma
216. Ghost
217. Food

Ten stroke radicals
218. Tail
219. Tripod
220. Whisker

Eleven stroke radicals
221. Hemp
222. Deer

Twelve stroke radicals
223. Black

Thirteen stroke radicals
224. Drum
225. Rat

Fourteen stroke radicals
226. Nose

Steps in identifying the radical

As you become more familiar with looking at Chinese characters, you will begin to familiarize yourself of the various shapes which make up the 226 radicals. At first it will seem like any part of the character may potentially be the radical. However, radicals tend to appear in certain places.

First of all, look at the character for "good" (好). You should be able to see that it is a combination of two different design elements. There is a right and left character. In other words, it has right and left sides which exist independently of each other. Although combined, the right and left sides do not run into each other or touch when written in *kai shu*. Two out of every three Chinese characters are comprised of a right and left-hand side.

If you have a right and left sided character like the word *hao* or "good", the radical is usually the part on the left-hand side. This is not always the case, but it is a good rule of thumb to start from. Therefore, if you have a character made up of left and right hand sections, count the number of strokes necessary to write the left hand section. The left hand section in the word *hao* or "good" is written with three strokes. It is the female or woman radical. Therefore, you can find it under the column of three stroke radicals, number 73.

The commonly occurring radicals found on the left hand side are 8, 10, 21, 33, 40, 41, 42, 48, 49, 55, 57, 62, 68, 69, 71, 73, 74, 75, 77, 83, 85, 87, 88, 94, 97, 100, 103, 106, 110, 114, 118, 129, 133, 136, 141, 147, 148, 149, 150, 159, 163, 171, 174, 175, 176, 177, 182, 193, 196, 198, 200, 201, 202, 203, 206, 209, 211, 213, 215, 222, and 224. The ones that are underlined are the most commonly seen of these.

The radicals 17, 28, 32, 34, 56, 63, 113, 119, 120, 152, and 170 are generally found on the right-hand side of a two-sided character. In this case, the left-hand side is rarely a radical.

If you have a character where a potential radical seems to stretch from one side to the other of a character, as in the characters 后, 历, 远, 廷, 应, once again, the left-hand side is usually the radical. In the foregoing examples, the radicals are respectively numbers 22, 13, 47, 36, and 44.

Common radicals which stretch from left to right include 13, 14, 15, 22, 36, 38, 44, 47, 56, 67, 86, 127, 165, 173, and 189.

Other characters are divided into top and bottom sections. For instance, the word *ai*, mugwort (艾) has a top (⺿) and a bottom (乂). Usually, I recommend trying the top to see if it is the radical. The top part of the character *ai* is written with three strokes. Therefore, scan the three stroke radical column to see if you can find this radical. You should've found it as number 50, the grass radical. However, in some cases, the bottom part is the radical. When you see characters which have a (心) or the heart radical on the bottom or (灬), the fire radical underneath, always take these as the radical first. The heart radical is written with four strokes, so you will find it as number 81. The fire radical (there are two fire radicals; this one shows fire under a pot) also has four strokes. It is number 80. Just a little less than one quarter of Chinese characters have a top-bottom structure.

If a character has a top and bottom half *and both halves appear in the radical list*, then the lower half is usually the radical. For instance, in the characters 忈 and 盐, the radicals are respectively number 81 and 146. However, if you have a top-bottom character with 山, radical 60, on top, it is usually the radical. Radical 60 means mountain. Likewise, if you have a top-bottom character with 穴 on top, radical 128, it is usually the radical.

If a character seems to have a hat on top, then this hat or crown is usually the radical. For instance, the radicals in the following characters 六, 京, 每, 字, 艾, and 党 are 9, 9, 20, 45, 50, and 139. The common roof, hat, or crown radicals include 9, 18, 20, <u>45</u>, <u>50</u>, 92, 93, 134, and 139, with those that are underlined being the most common.

Yet other characters are written as if their contents were written within an enclosure. Look at radical number 59 (囗) under the three stroke column. It appears to be the same as radical number 58, just larger. Radical 59 describes a four-sided box which encompasses various forms written within it. In such characters, radical 59 is always the radical. Likewise, radical 46 (门), the gate radical, encloses various things within it. When you see radical 46 in a character, it is almost always the radical.

If a character is made up of three parts, such as the character 柴,, as in *Chai Hu*, Radix Bupleuri, the radical is typically the largest element. In this case, it is radical 94, wood or tree, at the bottom.

There are also a few very commonly seen radicals. Whenever you come across any of these, try them first before trying any other parts of the character as the radical. Some very common radicals when working with the Chinese medical literature are numbers 21 (亻), 58 (口), 81 (心), 118 (月), 40 (氵), 47 (辶), 94 (木), 55 (扌), 33 (阝), 50 (艹), 87 (王), and 92 (艹).

There are also a few radicals which are easily confused for each other by beginners. For instance, numbers 13 and 22 are very similar, but 22 has a slanted top section, whereas the top section of number 13 is horizontal. Number 65 and 113 look very similar. Number 65 is written with only three strokes, the top right angle being only a single stroke. In radical number 113, the horizontal line at the top is written by itself. Therefore 113 is written with a total of four strokes. Radicals 106 and 107 seem identical and both are written with four strokes. However, the right hand "leg" on number 107 curves up at the bottom, while on number 106 it is straight.

The above suggestions will help you find the radicals of 19 out of 20 characters. However, as in any language, there are exceptions. For instance, in the character 妾, both elements are radicals. Therefore, based on the above guidelines, we might think that the radical is number 73 (女). Alas, the radical is number 126 (立). In the character 耶, again both right and left sides are radicals. But instead of the radical being number 163 (耳), it is number 34 (阝).

And then there are some truly eccentric characters. For instance, the radical for 器 is 58 (口), not 96, while the radical for (求) is 1 (丶). How is the beginner going to know this? Bottom line: you're not. Then how are you going to identify the radical? Through trial and error. You just keep looking up the various parts of the character until you find the radical under which the character is listed in the Character Index.

If all else fails in terms of finding the radical, there are five "bail-out" techniques. The first is to consider the whole character as the radical. For instance, the radicals with larger numbers of strokes may often be taken as complex characters having radicals. Radicals number 210 (鱼), 211 (音), 212 (革), 213 (是), etc. all look like they are made up of different parts. However, they are radicals all by themselves. Therefore, if you have a complex character with a total of eight or more strokes and you cannot find it listed under any of the parts or pieces which are also radicals on their own, see if the whole character is a radical itself. As you get familiar with the Radical Index, you will automatically remember that some of these characters are radicals all by themselves.

Secondly, if you have tried and tried to find the radical and every attempt has ended in failure, don't forget number 227, the characters that don't have radicals. There are only a small number of these, and after you have been frustrated by looking them up a few times, you will tend to remember them automatically. Of course, if you have the time and inclination, it certainly doesn't hurt to memorize this list of 11 characters.

The third bail-out option is to us a "cheat sheet" in the back of *Matthew's Chinese English Dictionary*. This is the most commonly used Chinese-English dictionary for complicated characters in academe. It can usually be found at college bookstores at colleges which teach Chinese. On page 1222 of *Matthew's*, there begins an index titled, "List of Characters Having Obscure Radicals." If you can't find the radical in a character, you can always try going to this index. In this case, you count the *total number of strokes* and look down the index to the list of characters with that number strokes. When you find the character in this index, there will be an Arabic number to the right of it which is the page number on which this character can be found in *Matthew's*. By going to that page, you can at least find out the meaning of the word, even though you still will not know what the radical is and how to look it up in your Pinyin, simplified character Chinese-English dictionary. Take heart, one twelfth of all characters in *Matthew's* are listed in this section on characters having obscure radicals.

A fourth method is to scan the Character Index under the first seven or so radicals. These are all one and two stroke radicals. When they are used, the way they are written is sometimes modified or they actually cross through other strokes. So they may not appear as free-standing components but are integrated more contiguously into the character than most radicals. Basically, we are talking about scanning down, column by column, a half page of characters. An extension of this is to scan the entire Character Index. Although this is a bit extreme, if you do persist in trying to translate, it is a fair wager that you will resort to this technique at least once out of desperation.

And the fifth bail-out technique is to ask a native Chinese speaker. It may be the character you are looking for has something peculiar about it which only a native speaker knows. However, when you do this and even the Chinese person cannot find the radical for the character in question, this will put your own frustrations in a more humane perspective!

6
How to Look Up a Chinese Character

Once you've found what you think is the radical in the Radical Index of your Chinese-English dictionary, make note of its number, *i.e.*, the number of the radical. Next, count the total number of strokes in *the remainder of the character.* Let's take the character *gan* (肝) as an example. It is a left and right character, meaning it has right and left-hand sections. The left-hand section is written with four strokes, remembering that the upper right-hand corner is a single stroke. If we look under the four stroke column in the Radical Index, we will find this shape under radical number 118, the "meat" or "moon" radical. Next we count the number of strokes remaining. There are three strokes to the right-hand section of the character.

With this information in hand, we turn to the Character Index which follows the Radical Index. There we'll see columns headed by Arabic numbers in parentheses. These Arabic numbers in parentheses are the numbers of the radicals. Therefore, we need to turn to column (118). Now we are where all the characters whose radical is number 118 are listed. Looking under (118), we again see the characters for two strokes (二画), three strokes (三画), four strokes (四画), etc. The *remaining number* of strokes of the character we are trying to look up is three. Therefore, we should look down the column until we find the section of characters with the meat or moon radical written with three remaining strokes.

As it so happens, we get a match for the character we are looking for in the very first character in the list under three strokes. To the right of the character there are again some Arabic numerals. In this case 218. This is the page number on which the character we are looking for can be found. Now we must turn to page 218 and scan the page for our character. There are two columns on the page and there are larger, bold faced (*i.e.*, darker colored) characters on the left-hand sides of these two columns. We need to scan these larger and darker colored characters till we find the character we are looking for. Bingo! The character we are looking for means liver, one of the five viscera of Chinese medicine.

Therefore, the steps in looking up a Chinese character in a Chinese-English dictionary are:

1. Identify the radical by counting its strokes and finding it in the Radical Index.
2. Turn to that number radical in the Character Index.
3. Count the remaining number of strokes in the character.
4. Scan the list of characters under that number of strokes under that radical.
5. Turn to the page number listed next to the character under that number of strokes under that radical.
6. Scan the large, bold-faced characters on the left of the columns on that page until you find the character you are looking for.
7. Read the definition.

OK, this is not as easy as looking up a word in an English dictionary. That being said, get over it! Although this is a cumbersome, time-consuming, seven step method, it's the only way you can look up the English meaning of a Chinese character if you do not know its Pinyin spelling. If you do know its Pinyin spelling, then you can look the character up alphabetically by scanning the several pages with all those characters with that Pinyin spelling. If you know the character's tone, then you can go directly to the characters with that tone.

Practice, practice, practice!

Like any skill, the skill of looking up a Chinese character in a Chinese-English dictionary is one which gets better with practice. The more you practice, the better you will become at A) identifying radicals, and B) counting the remaining strokes. Therefore, let's practice looking up some characters. (If you just read this section and do not actually go through all the steps with your dictionary, you will not develop the skills necessary to translate modern medical Chinese. So, please, do the exercises; don't just skim!)

First, let's look up the character 易. This character has a top and bottom half. We've seen the top half before (日). Maybe it's the radical. Count the number of strokes.

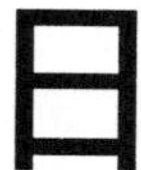

Yes, this part is written with four strokes, remembering that the top right-hand corner of a box is always written with a single joined stroke. Now find this potential radical in the Radical Index under the column of radicals with four strokes (四画). You'll see two which look very similar: 103 & 104. The difference is that 104 is more horizontal. It is used less often as a radical. So, let's assume that the radical is 103. Turn to the Character Index and find radical 103. Next, count the remaining number of strokes.

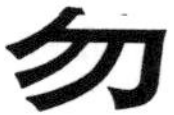

Again four strokes. Go to the four stroke column under radical 103 and scan down the list of characters with this radical plus four strokes. It is just one character more than halfway down this list. On its right is an Arabic number. That is the page on which this character's English definition is found. Turn to that page and scan the page, looking at the larger, bold-faced characters on the left-hand sides of the columns.

You should have found that this character's very first meaning is "easy". See—this is easy! It is not impossible. This character also means change as in the 易经, *or Yi Jing (The Classic of Change)*. It's just a different way of looking up a word based on the logic of the Chinese language, not on the logic of English.

Now let's look up 脾. It is a left and right-sided character. We said that if you have a right and left-sided character, the left side is usually the radical. So, count how many strokes there are in the left-hand side.

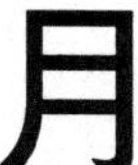

Right, there are four strokes. Therefore, look for this radical in the Radical Index in the column under four strokes (四画). You should now have found number 118. Do you remember that we have looked up this radical before? Now turn to radical 118 in the Character Index. Count the remaining number of strokes.

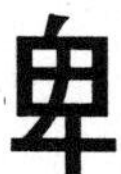

You should have counted eight strokes. Now look under the column of radical 118 with eight strokes (八画). The character is the next to the last one in that column. Find the page number to the right of that character and turn to that page. Scan that page to find the character. You should have found that the character is *pi* or spleen.

Next, let's look up the character 益. This character is a top and bottom character. If we count the top part, we get five strokes. If we look in the Radical Index under five strokes, however, there is no such radical. That means that the bottom part is the radical. This is also written with five strokes. If we look this up in the Radical Index under five strokes (五画), we find that this is a radical, number 146. Turn to radical number 146 in the Character Index and scan down under this radical plus five strokes. Remember, that is the number of strokes in the top part. In fact, the character we are looking for is the first one in the list. Now turn to the page number listed and what do we find? The word is *yi* and it means to benefit, profit, or advantage. It also means to increase. As we will see further on, Nigel Wiseman translates this word when it is used as a treatment principle as "to boost".

Exercise: Please look up the following Chinese medical characters. While "solving the problem", cover the answers. Then, after you think you have found the answers, uncover them and check how you did.

1. 针

A. The radical is on which side?
B. The radical has how many strokes?
C. The radical is number __________.
D. The remaining number of strokes is __________.
E. The word means __________________.

Answers: A. Left; B. 5; C. 147; D. 2; E. Needle, as in acupuncture

2. 灸

A. The radical is on the top or bottom?

B. The radical has how many strokes?
C. The radical number is _________.
D. The remaining number of strokes is ________.
E. The word means ____________________.

Answers: A. Bottom; B. 4; C. 83; D. 3; E. Moxibustion

3. 白

A. What is the radical?
B. The radical has how many strokes?
C. The radical number is _________.
D. The remaining number of strokes is _________.
E. The word means ___________.

Answers: A. Entire character; B. 5; C. 150; D. 0; E. White

The bottom part, radical 103 might have been the radical plus one stroke at the top, but it isn't. In this case, the whole thing is the radical. This character is part of the name of many Chinese medicinals, such as *Bai Shao* (Radix Albus Paeoniae Lactiflorae), *Bai Du* (Radix Stemonae), *Bai Guo* (Semen Gingkonis Bilobae), *Bai Mao Gen* (Rhizoma Imperatae Cylindricae), etc., etc.

4. 生

A. What is the radical?
B. How many strokes does the radical have?
C. The radical number is ___________.
D. The remaining number of strokes is ________.
E. The word means _________.

Answers: A. The little right to left sloping curve on the upper left-hand side; B. 1; C. 4; D. 4; E. Life, to be born, to arise, to engender

5. 道

A. What is the radical?
B. How many strokes does the radical have?
C. The radical number is _________.
D. The remaining number of strokes is ________.
E. The word means ___________.

Answers: A. The left-hand section which comes across to the right underneath; B. 3; C. 47; D. 9; path or way as in Daoism or the *Dao De Jing (Classic of the Way & Virtue)*

6. 和

A. What is the radical?
B. How many strokes does the radical have?
C. The radical number is ________.
D. The remaining number of strokes is ________.
E. The word means ______________.

Answers: The left-hand side; B. 5; C. 149; D. 3; E. Gentle, mild, harmonious, peace, together with

When you found this character in the character index, you should have seen that the same character was listed three or four times in a row with different page numbers after each listing. This means that this character has several different pronunciations and, therefore, several different meanings. In this case, you would have to look up the definitions of each of these and then decide on an *ad hoc* basis which fits better the meaning of the sentence you are trying to translate. We will discuss the issue of interpretation in a following chapter.

7. 实

A. What is the radical?
B. How many strokes does the radical have?
C. The radical number is ________.
D. The remaining number of strokes is ________.
E. The word means ____________.

Answers: A. The top part; B. 3; C. 45; D. 5; E. Replete

8. 寒

A. What is the radical?
B. How many strokes does the radical have?
C. The radical number is ________.
D. The remaining number of strokes is ________.
E. The word means ____________.

Answers: A. The top part; B. 3; C. 45; D. 9; E. Cold

9. 温

A. What is the radical?
B. How many strokes does the radical have?
C. The radical number is ________.
D. The remaining number of strokes is ________.
E. The word means ____________.

Answers: A. The left-hand section; B. 3; C. 40; D. 9; E. Warm

10. 保

A. What is the radical?
B. How many strokes does the radical have?
C. The radical number is _______.
D. The remaining number of strokes is _______.
E. The word means _________.

Answers: A. The left-hand side; B. 2; C. 21; D. 7; E. To protect or defend

11. 包

A. What is the radical?
B. How many strokes does the radical have?
C. The radical number is _______.
D. The remaining number of strokes is _______.
E. The word means _________.

Answers: A. The top part; B. 2; C. 26; D. 3; E. Wrapper, envelope

12. 病

A. What is the radical?
B. How many strokes does the radical have?
C. The radical number is _______.
D. The remaining number of strokes is _______.
E. The word means _________.

Answers: A. The left-hand part which extends over the top; B. 5; C. 127; D. 5; E. Disease

13. 法

A. What is the radical?
B. How many strokes does the radical have?
C. The radical number is _______.
D. The remaining number of strokes is _______.
E. The word means _________.

Answers: A. The left-hand section; B. 3; C. 40; D. 5; E. Method, technique

14. 防

A. What is the radical?
B. How many strokes does the radical have?
C. The radical number is _______.
D. The remaining number of strokes is _______.
E. The word means ___________.

Answers: A. Left-hand section; B. 2; C. 33; D. 4; E. Prevent

15. 补

A. What is the radical?
B. How many strokes does the radical have?
C. The radical number is _______.
D. The remaining number of strokes is _______.
E. The word means ___________.

Answers: A. The left-hand section; B. 5; C. 129; D. 2; E. Mend, patch, repair. Wiseman gives supplement when used as a Chinese medical principle.

16. 命

A. What is the radical?
B. How many strokes does the radical have?
C. The radical number is _______.
D. The remaining number of strokes is _______.
E. The word means ___________.

Answers: A. The top roof-like part; B. 2; C. 23; D. 6; Destiny or life

17. 真

A. What is the radical?
B. How many strokes does the radical have?
C. The radical number is _______.
D. The remaining number of strokes is _______.
E. The word means ___________.

Answers: A. The top cross; B. 2; C. 12; D. 8; E. True, real, genuine

18. 难

A. What is the radical?

B. How many strokes does the radical have?
C. The radical number is _______.
D. The remaining number of strokes is ________.
E. The word means ___________.

Answers: A. The left-hand section; B. 2; C. 35; D. 8; E. Difficult, as in 难经 or the *Nan Jing* (*The Classic of Difficulties*)

19. 阴

A. What is the radical?
B. How many strokes does the radical have?
C. The radical number is _______.
D. The remaining number of strokes is ________.
E. The word means ___________.

Answers: A. The left-hand section; B. 2; C. 33; D. 4; yin, as in yin and yang

20. 以

A. What is the radical?
B. How many strokes does the radical have?
C. The radical number is _______.
D. The remaining number of strokes is ________.
E. The word means ___________.

Answers: A. The right-hand section; B. 2; C. 23; D. 2; in order to

Some examples of characters with difficult radicals to identify

The following characters are all ones with which a beginner may have some difficulty. In fact, they are all characters which I have had some difficulty looking up when doing this or that Chinese medical translation. The main axiom of looking up characters in a Chinese-English dictionary is, "If at first you don't succeed, try, try again."

Mai (麦) as in *Mai Ya* (Tuber Ophiopogonis Japonici) is not under 韦 and it is not under 夂 . What to do after looking under both of those radicals? Try looking at the whole thing as a radical. It is radical number 188. When you turn to radical 188 in the Character Index, you will see that the first entry is not headed by any number of strokes. This is because there are no remaining strokes. So you would just look up the page number to the right of this character/radical.

Xian (涎) means saliva or drool. Its radical is easy to identify. It is on the left-hand side and has three strokes. This is the water radical, number 40. However, when you go to count the right-hand side, most non-Chinese will count eight strokes. Actually, it is written correctly with six.

Chou (丑) means something ugly or unsightly. However, it is also the second of the 12 earthly branches. Where's the radical? It has only one stroke. It is radical number 2 (一). One approach to finding this character is to scan the lists of characters under the first several, very simple one and two stroke radicals.

Shu (鼠) means rat or mouse. It is a character with lots of strokes and none of them immediately jump out as the radical. So count all of the strokes, in this case, 13, and see if the whole character is a radical. It is.

La (辣) means hot, spicy, or peppery. It is a left-right character. Its radical is the part on the left. This radical is written with seven strokes. It is radical number 186. However, when joined to 束, the bottom section is written so that it turns to the left. Beginners are apt not to see this shape as essentially the same as number 186 in the radical index. Likewise, radicals number 23, 24, 27, 42, 79, 110, 116, 157, 166, 178, and 184 are frequently written slightly differently than they look in the Radical Index when combined with other elements to make up more complex characters. When you look at these radicals in the Radical Index, you will see that each one of these has two forms, the one appearing in parentheses being more how the radical looks when it is used in combination as opposed to when it is used as its own word.

Cheng (乘) means to ride, take advantage of, or multiply. The radical is number 149 with five strokes. Can you see that radical embedded within the complexity of the character altogether? Then there are five strokes remaining.

Fan (反) means to turn over, opposite, or on the contrary. The radical is the part on the left which reaches over the top to the right. If you looked under radical number 13 with two strokes, the number of strokes was correct, but you have the wrong radical. Actually, its radical is number 22. Its top line slants upward to the right, while number 13 has a purely horizontal top.

Jia (佳) means good, fine, beautiful. Its radical is number 21 with two strokes on the left-hand side. However, when you go to count up the remaining strokes, if you tried to find the character under five strokes, it isn't there. That's because the remaining portion of the character on the right-hand side is not written with a single vertical stroke down the center. Rather, this part of the character is made up of two *tu* (土) or earth characters stacked one on top of the other. Therefore, the remaining number of strokes is six.

Chao (朝) means court, government, or dynasty. It is a left and right-sided character. We've already looked up the right-hand portion twice previously. So we know that that symbol can be a radical. However, if we look up radical 118 with a remainder of eight strokes, we do not find the character we are looking for. So now, try seeing if the left-hand side is a radical. It is. It is number 203, and eight stroke radical. That means the remaining strokes are four. So we will find this character under radical 203 plus four strokes.

Qi (器) means implement or utensil. It is a complex character made up of four boxes at the four corners and a character in the middle of these. The character in the middle is written with four strokes and is radical number 96. The problem is that number 96 is not this character's radical.

Rather it is number 58, a three stroke radical. Therefore, subtract three strokes and count all the remaining strokes. Then look under radical 58 plus 13 strokes. *Voilà!*

Cai (才) means ability or talent. Altogether it has three strokes. It is not really a left-right character nor a top-bottom character. Its radical is the one stroke radical, number 2. Then there are two strokes remaining.

Mie (灭) means to extinguish. It shows a picture of putting a lid on top of fire. The radical could either be the top horizontal stroke, radical number 2, or it could be the four stroke fire radical, number 83. In actual fact, it is number 83. That means you would look this character up in the Character Index under radical 83 with one remaining stroke.

Jiu (就) means in regard to. It appears to be a straightforward left-right character. The problem is that neither the left nor right side components are radicals in and of themselves. As it turns out, the radical is the two strokes on top of the left hand side, radical number 9. Then there are 10 strokes remaining.

Wang (忘) means to neglect or forget. It is a character with a top and a bottom. Previously, I said that when you see a top-bottom character and there is the heart radical (心), number 81, on the bottom to always try that first as the radical. Well, usually that is a good idea. However, in this particular case, it doesn't work. The radical is the three stroke radical at the top, number 43.

Bi (必) means certainly, surely, necessarily. It does not seem to have either a top or bottom, left or right. Three out of four of its strokes look like the heart radical (心), number 81, we just discussed above. In that case, there would be one remaining stroke through the center of the heart. However, when we look under radical 81, there's no such character under one stroke. So we try again. That single stroke could be the radical. In that case it would be radical number 4. We look up radical number 4 plus three strokes and we still do not see our character listed. What to do? We go to the very beginning of the character index, starting with radical number one. There are so few characters listed under number 1 that they are not separated by numbers of strokes. Rather, they are all listed in order from least to most strokes. Sure enough, sitting in the middle of this list is the character we are looking for and the page number on which we will find its definition.

What you find when you look a character up

Let's say you have looked up the character 采 (*cai*, to pick, pluck, gather). Below is a reproduction of what you will see.

cǎi

采　cǎi　① pick; pluck; gather: ～茶 pick tea/ ～药 gather medicinal herbs/ ～珍珠 dive for pearls ② mine; extract: ～煤 mine coal/ ～油 extract oil ③ adopt; select: ～取一系列措施 adopt a series of measures ④ complexion; spirit: 兴高～烈 in high spirits
另见 cài

On the left-hand side, you will see the character printed in bold face and a larger font followed by its Pinyin romanization and tone mark. In this case, the tone mark indicates this word is pronounced with the third tone. Next comes an Arabic number 1 in a circle (①) followed by the words "pick; pluck; gather". Then comes a colon. After the colon there is a tilde (~) followed by the character 茶 (*cha*). This character means "tea". The tilde is meant to represent the character we have looked up. In effect, ~ (*cha*) means 采茶 (*cai cha*), "to pick tea". This phrase is followed by another tilde and the character 药 (*yao*). *Yao* means "medicinal". So 采药 , *cai yao* means "to pick or gather medicinals". Again there is a tilde followed by the characters 珍珠(*zhen zhu*) which mean "pearl/pearls". Therefore, 采珍珠, *cai zhen zhu* means "to gather or dive for pearls". Next we see an Arabic number 2 in a circle (②). Following this are two more verbs, "to mine" and "to extract". Therefore, when the word *cai* precedes the words for coal, together they mean "to mine coal", while if the word *cai* precedes the word for oil, they mean "to extract oil". Then we see an Arabic number 3 in a circle (③). Following it are the words "to adopt" or "select". Therefore, when the word *cai* precedes the characters following the tilde in the example, these words together mean "to adopt a series of measures". And finally we come to an Arabic number 4 in a circle (④) followed by the words "complexion" and "spirit". When the word *cai* is used in the following phrase, where the word *cai* is symbolized by the tilde, this phrase means "high spirits".

Therefore, each set of words following an Arabic number in a circle is a different meaning or usage of the word under discussion. In one situation, the word *cai* means "to pluck, pick, or gather". In another, it means "mine" or "extract". In another, it means "to adopt or select", and in yet a fourth, it means "complexion" or "spirit". Therefore, when it comes to translating this word, we will have to decide, based on the other words it is combined with, which of these four English meanings are the right one in a given passage. We will discuss further how you pick the right meaning from those given under a word in a dictionary below. However, this is a skill I have not yet figured out how to really teach. As we will see below, it takes both logic and intuition.

Under the four definitions of the word *cai*, we also see two other characters: 另见 (*ling jian*). They mean, "also see." These are then followed by the Pinyin *cai*. This means that there are two different words written the same way, yet pronounced differently. In this case, the Pinyin vowels and consonants are the same, but the tone is different. However, in other cases, the vowels and consonants may be quite different. If we have not found a meaning under those definitions given above, then we must turn in our Pinyin Chinese-English dictionaries to the page where this other word is given. In this particular case, the character is on the next page.

cài

采 cài
另见 cǎi
【采邑】 càiyì   fief; benefice

It does not give any definition but merely says to also see the *cai* we have just been looking at. However, it does go on to give a compound term, 采邑(*cai yi*), fief, benefice. Therefore, whenever you come to the bottom of the definitions of a word and you see the characters 另. . . ,

i.e., also____, you need to turn to that same character under a different Pinyin spelling and check to see if the definition which works in the line you are reading is one of those.

7
Let's Give Translating a Try

In chapter 9 below, I talk about what I think you should try to read first. But before we go on to that, let's try to do a little translation. Most Western practitioners of Chinese medicine begin their study and prescription of Chinese formulas with so-called patent medicines. These patent medicines usually have both Chinese and English written on their boxes. Because the Chinese text is usually so short and succinct and because the Chinese texts and their English "translations" are usually at such variance, trying to read these labels is both an easy way to practice translation and a valuable insight the typical technical insufficiency of non-native English-speaker translations. Simply by reading the Chinese labels yourselves, you should gain a much better, clearer, more focused understanding of the clinical functions and indications of these patent medicines.

Below are reproductions of the outer packaging of several commonly used Chinese patent medicines. All these are written mainly in simplified characters. Because many Chinese patents produced in the PRC are made for export to overseas Chinese communities, the information on many Chinese patent medicines is printed with complex or traditional characters.

When you look at the above right panel from this Chinese patent medicine box, you will notice four large characters in the center. That is the name of the medicine; so let's start there. 前 (*qian*) means in front of or before. 列(*lie*) means to 1) arrange, to line up, sort, 2) to list, 3) to file, rank, or put in a row, and 4) kind or type. 腺 (*xian*) means gland. So we are talking about a gland. In traditional Chinese medicine, we have no glands. That means we probably should go directly to our Chinese-English medical dictionary. Front row gland, front list gland, front arranged gland all don't immediately make much sense. Front positioned gland makes a little more

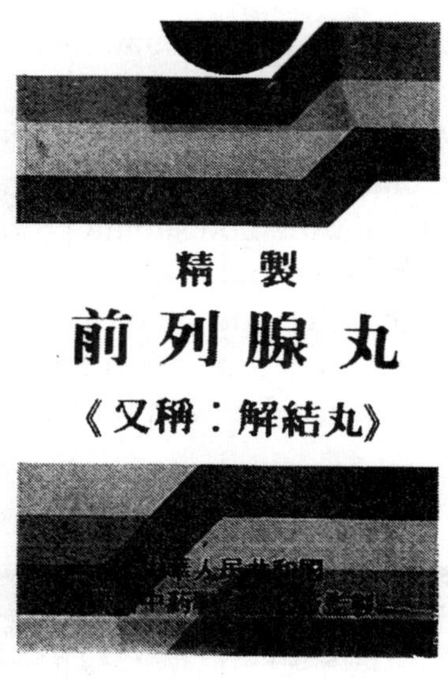

sense if you could then put that in Latin. But let's say you don't know any Latin. If you don't have a Chinese-English medical dictionary, go back to the word *qian* in your regular Pinyin Chinese-English dictionary and see if there are any compound terms with these three characters. Bingo! There is—prostate gland. Now try to find the fourth character. It is a radical all by itself. It is written with three strokes. It is radical number 66. Look up radical number 66 in the Character Index and turn to the page it is on in your dictionary. *Violà* It means pill. Therefore, the name of this patent medicine translates as "Prostate Gland Pills." For now, let's not worry about the characters underneath this name. They are written in complex characters. They read, "Also called: Resolving Binding Pills (*Jie Jie Wan*)."

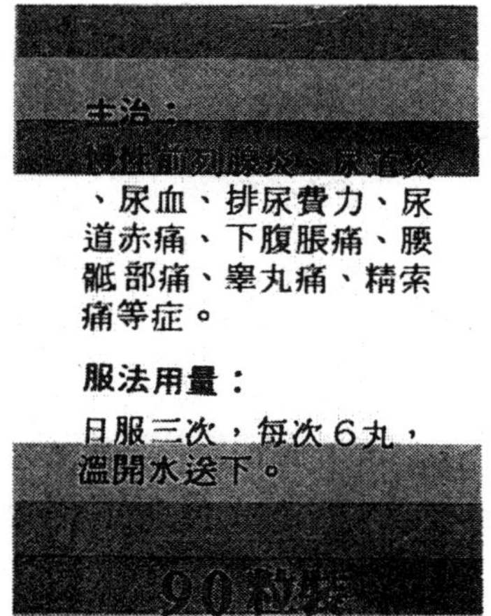

Exercise: Let's now turn to the panel on the left. Please try and translate the Chinese you see here. There are a couple of complicated characters, but I think you will be surprised how much you can translate even without being able to translate these few complicated characters. After you have translated this panel, compare your translation with mine below.

Bob's translation:

Mainly treats: Chronic prostatitis, urinary tract inflammation, bloody urine, expulsion of urine without force, urinary tract red and painful, lower abdominal distention and pain, low back and sacral area pain, testicular pain, and essence rope pain, *i.e.*, sperm cord pain

Administration method & use amount, *i.e.*, dosage: Daily take three times, each time six pills.

Although there were a couple of complex characters you might not have been able to find in your dictionary and the character 睾 (*gao*) is also a difficult one to look up, I bet you were still able to translate most of the above. You should probably write down somewhere that 睾丸 (*gao wan*) means testes. In fact, you should start keeping a notebook where you write down the meanings of hard-to-find characters. Just the act of writing these down will help you remember them. Even if you don't actually remember the meaning the next time you see this character, you are likely to remember that you had trouble with it before and that its meaning is written in your notebook.

Let's try another one.

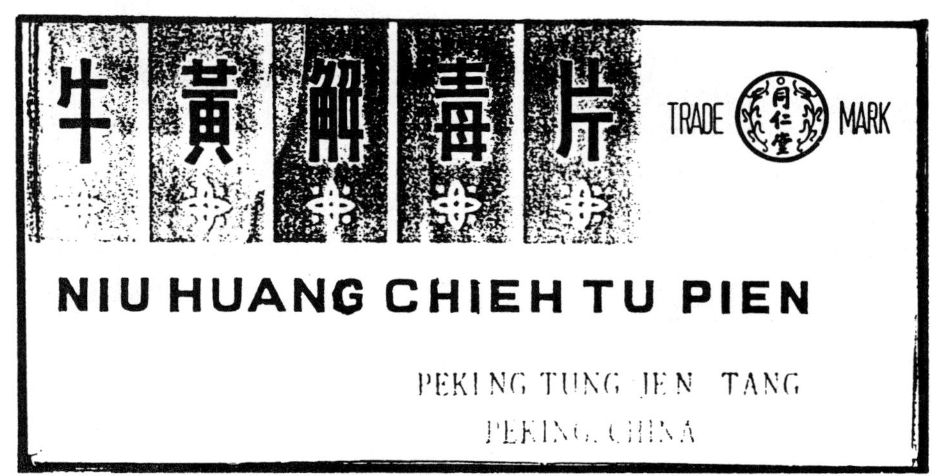

The top panel of this patent medicine box makes our life a little easier. Underneath the Chinese characters, their romanization is given. It's given in Wade-Giles, but you can easily transpose this into Pinyin by using Appendix 1 in the back of this workbook.

Exercise: After doing that, I recommend that you look up each word in the name of this medicine in your Pinyin Chinese-English dictionary. After you have done so, check the "answers" below.

Answers: *Niu* means cow or ox. *Huang* means yellow. So literally, *niu huang* means cow yellow. However, this is the proper name of a Chinese medicinal. If you scan the alphabetized Pinyin list of Chinese medicinals given in chapter 15, you will see it is Calculus Bovis or Cow Bezoar. *Jie* means to untie or unknot. Nigel Wiseman's translation of this character as a Chinese medical technical term is to resolve. *Du* means toxins. Therefore, *jie du* means to resolve toxins. *Pian* means slice, but it also means tablet. If we put this all together, we get, "Cow Bezoar Resolve Toxins Tablets."

Now look at the panel underneath. There is a Chinese text on top with its translation underneath.

> **主治：** 头痛眩晕，咽喉肿痛，胃火口疮，牙根出血，暴发火眼，咽痛发颐，耳痛鼻肿，风火牙痛，小儿内热，停食停乳，呕吐结滞。
>
> **Indications:**
> Headache, vertigo, sore throat, gastric fever, mouth pimples, gum-bleeding, acute ophthalmia, acute dysphagia, mumps, earache, toothache, children's fever, anorexia, nausea.

Exercise: Please translate this Chinese text. Then check your translation with mine and the one on the box.

Bob's translation:

Mainly treats (or indications): Head pain, *i.e.*, headache, dizziness and vertigo (or simply dizziness), throat swelling and pain, stomach fire mouth sores, teeth roots, *i.e.*, gums, exiting blood (or simply bleeding), sudden outbreak of red eyes, throat pain, *i.e.*, sore throat , expanded cheeks, ear pain, *i.e.*, earache, nasal swelling, wind fire tooth pain (or ache), pediatric internal heat, collected (but also means stopped) food, collected breast (milk), vomiting, binding and stagnation.

If you are a clinical practitioner of Chinese medicine, I think you will agree that there is more clinically useful information in my translation than in the Western medicalized gloss provided by the Chinese translator.

Let's do another.

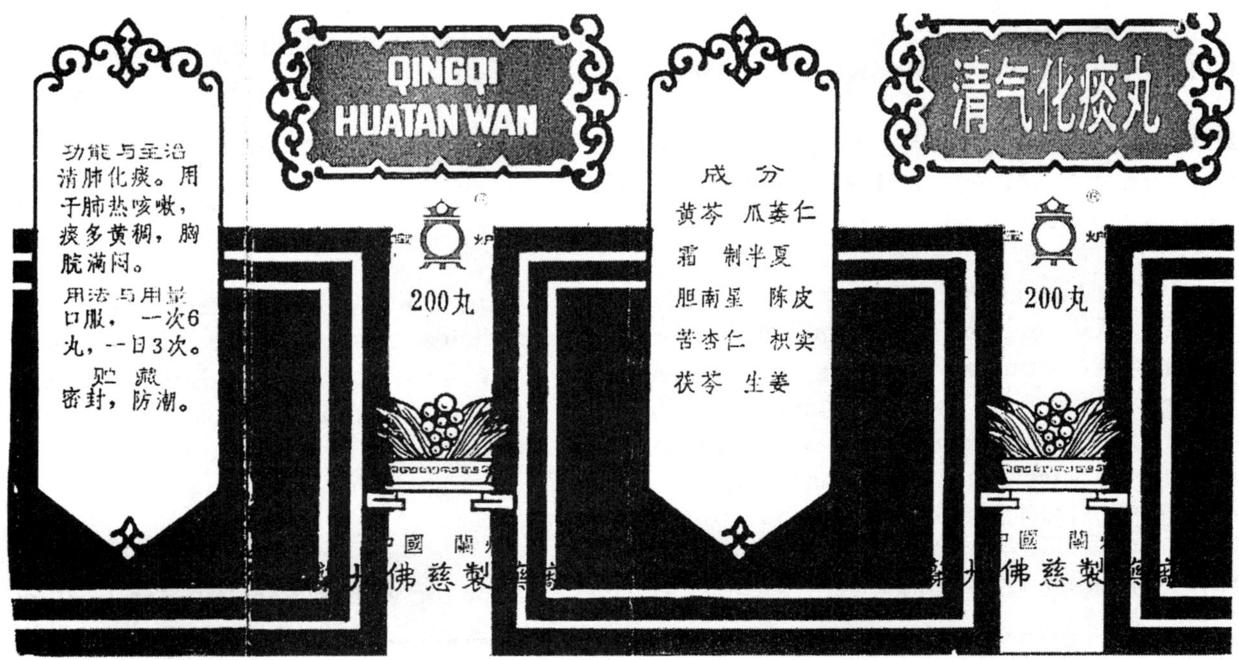

Above you will see the name of a common formula in Chinese medicine: *Qing Qi Hua Tan Wan*, Clear Qi & Transform Phlegm Pills. Underneath the name, you will see that the package contains 200 丸 (*wan*), 200 pills. The small characters at the bottom are the name of the pharmaceutical company written in complex characters. So let's turn our attention to the central panel.

The top two characters (成 分, *cheng fen*), mean composition. But we don't have to translate this section. Why look up every character in a list if there is some place you can check that list quickly against? When you see the word composition and then see a list of two or three character terms, you can immediately be fairly sure that these are the list of this formula's ingredients. You then can go look up these ingredients in an English language book, such as *Handbook of Chinese Herbs & Formulas, Vol. II* by Yeung Him-che or in Bensky & Barolet's *Formulas & Strategies*, where the ingredients of standard formulas are given in Latin, Pinyin, and Chinese characters. This is the "crafty", time-saving thing to do.

Exercise: Please translate the far left panel. After you have done so, check your translation against mine. You should be able to find all these characters.

Bob's translation:

Functions & indications (mainly treats): Clears the lungs and transforms phlegm. Used for lung heat cough, profuse, thick, yellow phlegm, chest and stomach duct fullness and oppression.

Method of use and dosage used: Take orally, one time six pills, one day three times. *I.e.,* take orally six pills each time, three times per day.

Storage: Keep sealed and prevent flooding or soaking.

Let's do one more.

Looking at the front of this patent
medicine box, right away we are faced with a slight
difficulty. The name of the medicine is printed in a
decorative script form. So here's the characters in
kai shu: 川贝精 (*chuan bei jing*). That means
Fritillaria Essence (or Extract). Underneath that are
the three characters 糖衣片 (*tang yi pian*). This says,
"Sugar-coated Pills."

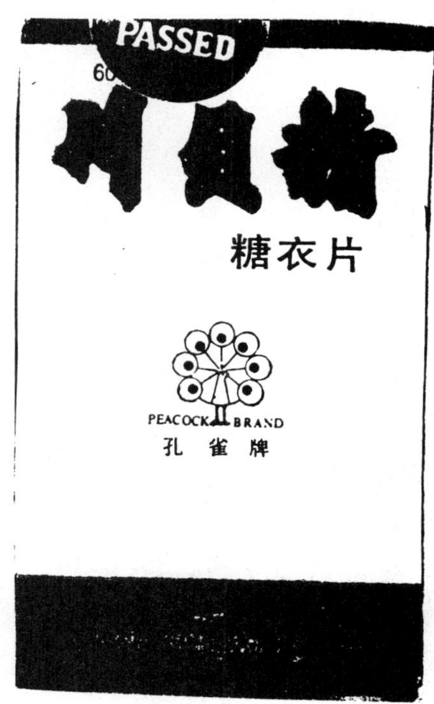

Exercise: Having been given that much, now you
translate the side panel. When you're done, check
your translation against mine.

Bob's translation:

Functions: Stops cough and transforms phlegm

Mainly treats (or indications): Acute and chronic
bronchitis, wind cold cough, etc.

Administration method: Each (time) take 3-6 tablets.

Hopefully, under 支 , *zhi*, you noticed that there is
the compound term *zhi qi guan* (支气管), bronchus.
Don't forget to always check for these compound terms.
They can save you a lot of time and trouble. Otherwise,
zhi, propping up, protruding, sustaining, or paying, may
have caused you some headaches. However, once you know
that the term, *zhi qi guan*, means bronchus or bronchi,
branching qi tubes makes sense retrospectively.

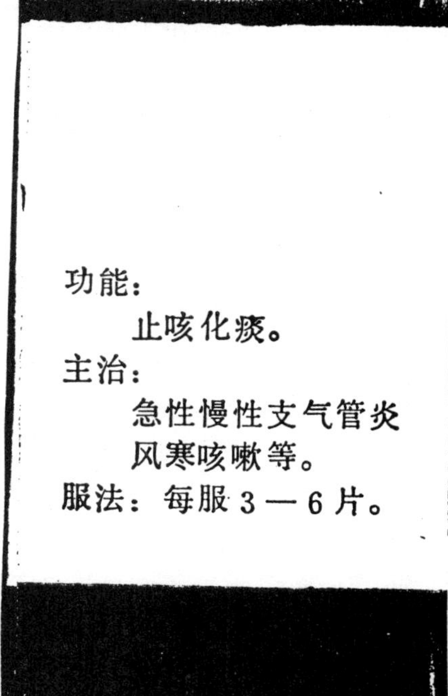

8
Let's Try Translating Some More

In the previous chapter, we did some very simple but nonetheless useful translations. Either there was no grammar or it was extremely simple. Hopefully you saw how much information you could extract simply by looking each character up in your Chinese-English dictionary. Below are some sections from modern Chinese medical books. I think you will find them both easy to translate and clinically useful.

The first section comes from **内科病良方** (*Nei Ke Bing Liang Fang, Fine Formulas for Internal Medicine Diseases*) by He Yuan-lin *et al.*, Yunnan University Press, Kunming, 1991, p. 55.

二、神志 病方

8. 治心烦、嗜睡、郁证

（1） **处方**：栀子10克　豆豉10克
　　　　 用法：水煎服。
　　　　 备注：治外感热病心烦不安者。

（2） **处方**：栀子10克　豆豉10克　甘草6克
　　　　 用法：水煎服。
　　　　 备注：治外感热病心烦不安而少气者。

（3） **处方**：栀子10克　豆豉10克　生姜10克
　　　　 用法：水煎服。
　　　　 备注：治外感热病心烦不安而兼呕者。

（4） **处方**：栀子10克　厚朴10克　枳实10克
　　　　 用法：水煎服。
　　　　 备注：治伤寒下后，心烦腹满，卧起不安者。

（5） **处方**：甜瓜蒂3克　赤小豆6克　山栀6克
　　　　 用法：水二杯，煮取一杯，先服半杯，得吐，止后
　　　　　　　　 服，不吐，再服。

· 55 ·

备注：治太阴温病，得之二、三日，心烦不安，痰涎壅
盛，胸中痞塞，欲呕者。虚者加人参芦 5 克。

（6）　处方：党参12克　麦冬12克　竹茹10克　半夏 6 克
茯苓 6 克　甘草 6 克　浮小麦10克
用法：水煎，分二次服。
备注：治病后余热不净，虚烦不安。

（7）　处方：党参12克　麦冬15克　五味子10克　生地15克
枣仁12克　茯神12克
用法：水煎，分三次服。
备注：治入夜心烦不安，口燥咽干。

（8）　处方：木通10克　生地12克　黄连 6 克　甘草 6 克
竹叶 6 克　水灯芯10克
用法：水煎，分三次服。
备注：治心中烦热，小便赤涩者。

（9）　处方：陈皮 6 克　半夏10克　茯苓10克　甘草 6 克
枳实10克　竹茹10克　黄连 6 克　芦根10克
麦冬10克　生姜 6 克
用法：水煎，分三次服。
备注：治心胸烦热而呕者。

Exercise: Please try to translate the above pages. After you are done, check your translation against mine below.

Bob's translation:

2. Mental-emotional Disease Formulas

8.　(For) the treatment (of) heart vexation, addiction to sleep (or somnolence), depression condition

(1)　Prescription (or Rx): Fructus Gardeniae Jasminoidis (*Zhi Zi*), 10g, Semen Praeparatum Sojae (*Dou Chi*), 10g

Use method (or method of use): Decoct in water and take (orally).

Remarks: Treats external affection heat disease heart vexation and disquietude (or restlessness, lack of calm).

(2)   Rx: Fructus Gardeniae Jasminoidis (*Zhi Zi*), 10g, Semen Praeparatum Sojae (*Dou Chi*), 10g, Radix Glycyrrhizae (*Gan Cao*), 6g

Method of use: Decoct in water and take.

Remarks: Treats external affection heat disease heart vexation and disquietude and reduced qi.

(3)   Rx: Fructus Gardeniae Jasminoidis (*Zhi Zi*), 10g, Semen Praeparatum Sojae (*Dou Chi*), 10g, uncooked Rhizoma Zingiberis (*Sheng Jiang*), 10g

Method of use: Decoct in water and take.

Remarks: Treats external affection heat disease heart vexation and disquietude with simultaneous vomiting

(4)   Rx: Fructus Gardeniae Jasminoidis (*Zhi Zi*), 10g, Cortex Magnoliae Officinalis (*Hou Po*), 10g, Fructus Immaturis Citri Aurantii (*Zhi Shi*), 10g

Method of use: Decoct in water and take.

Remarks: Treats damage by cold afterwards (or sequelae), heart vexation, abdominal fullness, disquietude (when) lying down (or) standing.

(5)   Rx: Pediculus Cucumidis Melonis (*Tian Gua Di*), 3g, Semen Phaseoli Calcarati (*Chi Xiao Dou*), 6g, Fructus Gardeniae Jasminoidis (*Shan Zhi*), 6g

Method of use: Take two cups of water and boil down to one cup. First administer a half cup. [After] obtaining vomiting, stop later administration. (If) there is no vomiting, administer again.
Remarks: Treats *tai yin* warm disease going on for two or three days, heart vexation and disquietude, phlegm drool congestion and exuberance, glomus and obstruction in the chest and middle (alternate reading: glomus and obstruction within the chest), desire to vomit.(For those with) vacuity, add the top (or crown) of Radix Panacis Ginseng (*Ren Shen Lu*), 5g.

(6)   Rx: Radix Codonopsitis Pilosulae (*Dang Shen*), 12g, Tuber Ophiopogonis Japonici (*Mai Dong*), 12g, Caulis Bambusae In Taeniis (*Zhu Ru*), 10g, Rhizoma Pinelliae Ternatae (*Ban Xia*), 6g, Sclerotium Poriae Cocos (*Fu Ling*), 6g, Radix Glycyrrhizae (*Gan Cao*), 6g, Fructus Levis Tritici Aestivi (*Fu Xiao Mai*), 10g

Method of use: Decoct in water and administer in two divided times (or doses).

Remarks: Treats the after(math) of disease (when) heat remains which has not been completely cleared away, vacuity vexation and disquietude.

(7)   Rx: Radix Codonopsitis Pilosulae (*Dang Shen*), 12g, Tuber Ophiopogonis Japonici (*Mai Dong*), 15g, Fructus Schisandrae Chinensis (*Wu Wei Zi*), 10g, uncooked Radix Rehmanniae (*Sheng Di*), 15g, Semen Zizyphi Spinosae (*Zao Ren*), 12g, Sclerotium Pararadicis Poriae Cocos (*Fu Shen*), 12g

Method of use: Decoct in water and administer in three divided doses.

Remarks: Treats entering night heart vexation and disquietude, oral dryness and dry throat.

(8)   Rx: Caulis Akebiae (*Mu Tong*), 10g, uncooked Radix Rehmanniae (*Sheng Di*), 12g, Rhizoma Coptidis Chinensis (*Huang Lian*), 6g, Radix Glycyrrhizae (*Gan Cao*), 6g, Folium Bambusae (*Zhu Ye*), 6g, Medulla Junci Effusi (*Shui Deng Xin*), 10g

Method of use: Decoct in water and administer in three divided doses.

Remarks: Treats heart and middle vexatious heat, inhibited voidings of reddish urine

(9)   Rx: Pericarpium Citri Reticulatae (*Chen Pi*), 6g, Rhizoma Pinelliae Ternatae (*Ban Xia*), 10g, Sclerotium Poriae Cocos (*Fu Ling*), 10g, Radix Glycyrrhizae (*Gan Cao*), 6g, Fructus Immaturus Citri Aurantii (*Zhi Shi*), 10g, Caulis Bambusae In Taeniis (*Zhu Ru*), 10g, Rhizoma Coptidis Chinensis (*Huang Lian*), 6g, Rhizoma Phragmitis Communi (*Lu Gen*), 10g, Tuber Ophiopogonis Japonici (*Mai Dong*), 10g, uncooked Rhizoma Zingiberis (*Sheng Jiang*), 6g

Method of use: Decoct in water and administer in three divided doses.

Remarks: Treats heart chest vexatious heat and vomiting.

When translating the above, you had to look at various lists or glossaries of Chinese medicinal names and identifications. You saw that certain Chinese medicinals may have more than a single name, for instance Medulla Junci Effusi, or that some Chinese medicinals have various contractions or abbreviations, such as Fructus Gardeniae Jasminoidis. You also saw that you often had to add words to the typically terse Chinese in order to make it read right in English. And you saw that sometimes you had to change the literal meaning of the Chinese word in order to make a typically English-sounding phrase or term. The above pages come from a formula compendium book, a whole genre within the Chinese medical literature. Hopefully, you can see that you could gain access to this entire genre fairly quickly and fairly easily.

The next section comes from 中国针灸方学 (*Zhong Guo Zhen Jiu Fang Xue, A Study of Chinese Acupuncture & Moxibustion Formulas*) by Xiao Shao-qing, Ningxia People's Press, Yinchuan, 1986, p. 347.

第十八节　小儿发热

一、解表清热方

【处方】

大椎ⅰ　外关ⅰ　少商↓　合谷ⅰ。

【主治】

外感发热：发热无汗，怕冷，鼻鸣，鼻流清涕，微咳，头痛，身痛，脉浮，指纹浮赤。热盛者多烦躁不安，或昏睡谵语。

【随症加穴】

身热无汗者，加复溜ⅰ；

烦躁不安者，加少府ⅰ；

昏睡谵语者，加中冲↓。

【方义】

本方具有解表清热的作用。取大椎、外关、合谷以解表退热；取少商刺血，以清肃肺热。若烦躁不安，昏睡谵语，此为里热盛而邪入心包，故取少府、中冲以清心宁神。

【穴效考证】

1·大椎：《甲乙经》说："伤寒热盛烦呕，大椎主之。"《类经图翼》说："窦太师治诸虚，寒热灸此。"

2·外关：《杂病穴法歌》说："一切风寒暑湿邪，头痛发热外关起。"《兰江赋》说："伤寒在表并头痛，外关泻动自然安。"

3·少商：《类经图翼》说："宜以三棱针刺微出血，泄诸脏之热，不宜灸。"

4·合谷：《兰江赋》说："更有伤寒真妙诀，三阴须要刺阳经，无汗更将合谷补。"

Exercise: Please try to translate the first four sections on this page. When you are done, compare your translation with mine below.

Bob's translation:

Chapter 18: Pediatric Fever

1. Resolve the Exterior & Clear Heat Formula

Rx: *Da Zhui* (GV 14), *Wai Guan* (TB 5), *Shao Shang* (Lu 11), *He Gu* (LI 4)

Mainly treats (or indications): External affection fever, fever with no sweating, fear of chill, nose noise (or noisy nose when breathing), runny nose which is clear and watery, slight cough, head pain (or headache), body pain, a floating pulse, finger veins floating (or superficial) and red. Heat exuberance mostly with vexation and agitation and disquietude, possible dizziness and delirious speech (while) asleep.

Following the condition added points:

For those with body heat (or generalized fever) but no sweating, add *Fu Liu* (Ki 7).

For those with vexation and agitation and disquietude (or restlessness), add *Shao Fu* (Ht 8).

For those with dizziness and delirious speech during sleep, add *Zhong Chong* (Per 9).

Formula idea or concept, *i.e.*, rationale: This formula has the effect of resolving the exterior and clearing heat. *Da Zhui, Wai Guan,* and *He Gu* are chosen in order to resolve the exterior and recede or abate heat or fever. *Shao Shang* is chosen and pierced to bleed in order to clear and depurate lung heat. If there is vexation and agitation and disquietude, dizziness, and delirious speech during sleep, this is due to interior heat exuberance and evils entering the pericardium. Therefore, *Shao Fu* and *Zhong Chong* are chosen to clear the heart and quiet the spirit.

What follows these first four sections is a section on cites concerning these points' efficacy. I'll leave these for you to translate if you'd like. However, since they come from premodern books and they are written in classical Chinese, they can be harder to translate. If you have gotten the acupuncture treatment you were looking for, you may not want to spend the time trying to decipher these literary quotes. I'm not saying that they're not good stuff, but they might not be the most advantageous use of your time and energy right now.

Here is one more page to try your hand translating. It is from 食物中药与便方 (*Shi Wu Zhong Yao Yu Bian Fang, Foods, Chinese Medicinals and Folk Formulas*) by Ye Ju-quan, Jiangsu Science & Technology Press, Nanjing, 1980, p. 227.

Exercise: Translate the following page. Begin with the page heading and then skip to the section headed 性味 (*xing wei*, nature [&] flavor[s]). Then compare your translation with mine below. (The section you're skipping tells us where grapes come from, that they can be eaten raw, dried into raisins, or made into wine. You know that, *and* it's not clinically very important.)

葡　　萄

Vitis vinifera L.

葡萄，属葡萄科植物。原产亚洲西部，现我国各地广为栽培，果可生食，制葡萄干和酿酒。藤及根供药用。果肉以栽培品为佳，药用多以野葡萄的藤及根为好。

〔性味〕甘、平、涩，无毒。

〔成分〕果含糖类，蛋白质，维生素B_1、B_2、C，菸酸及其他矿物质。根、茎及叶含橡胶质，糖类和酶等。

〔功用〕葡萄酒有营养强壮作用。根及藤祛风利水，治风痹筋骨痛，并有镇静、止呕、止痛作用。

〔便方〕1．怀孕呕吐或妊娠浮肿，小便不利：野葡萄根30克，水煎服。

2．肝炎，黄疸，风湿痛：鲜根30～90克，水煎服。

3．贫血，头晕心慌：葡萄酒适量饮服，一日2～3次。

4．风寒湿痹，筋骨疼痛，瘫痪麻木：葡萄根或藤、嫩桑枝、蚕砂各30克，加黄酒与水等量煎，一日2～3次分服。

5．跌打损伤，疼痛，风毒流痰（包括寒性脓疡，骨结核等）：葡萄根或藤60～90克，加酒、水合煎服，并以鲜根皮捣烂敷于患处。

Bob's translation:

Grapes

Nature & flavor: Sweet, level (or neutral), astringent, and without toxins

Composition: (We're going to skip this part too. Do you see B_1, B_2, and C? You should know from these that this section discusses the *Western* composition of grapes. We don't need to translate this. We could look this up in an English language nutrition book much faster and easier.)

Functions: Grape wine has a nutritious, strengthening effect. Its root and vine dispel wind and disinhibit water. They treat wind impediment sinew and bone pain. They also have settling and stilling, stopping vomiting, and stopping pain effects.

Folk formulas:

1. For vomiting during pregnancy or edema during pregnancy or inhibited urination: Wild Radix Viticis Viniferae (*Ye Pu Tao Gen*), 30g. Decoct in water and take (or administer).

2. Hepatitis, jaundice, wind damp (or rheumatic) pain: Decoct and take 30-90g of the fresh root in water and take.

3. Anemia, dizziness, heart fluster: Take a suitable amount of grape wine 2-3 times each day.

4. Wind cold damp impediment, sinew and bone aching and pain, paralysis and numbness: Take 30g each of Radix Seu Caulis Viticis Viniferae, tender Ramulus Mori Albi (*Sang Zhi*), and Excrementum Bombycis Mori (*Can Sha*), add equal amounts of yellow wine (*i.e.*, rice wine) and water, and boil. Take in 2-3 divided doses each day.

5. Injuries from falls, fractures, contusion, and strains (This is the gloss for this compound term in your dictionary. Literally it says falls, strikes, detriment, and damage.), aching and pain, wind toxins and flowing phlegm (including cold-natured pussy open sores, bone nodules, *i.e.*, tubercles, etc.): Take 60-90g of Radix Seu Caulis Viticis Viniferae, add wine and water, decoct, and take. Also apply the mashed fresh root bark to the affected area.

If you've done each of these three exercises, you have translated pages from books on Chinese "herbal" medicine, acupuncture-moxibustion, and Chinese dietary therapy. See, it's not so hard, and there's good, clinically useful information there. I also bet you are gaining a new understanding of the technical precision of Chinese medicine even from these few introductory exercises.

9
What to Translate

Before going on to discuss issues of interpretation, we must first identify the best things for beginners such ourselves to try to translate. Most Western neophytes make the mistake of trying to read the 内经 *(Nei Jing, Inner Classic),* 难经 *(Nan Jing, Classic of Difficulties),*伤寒论 *(Shang Han Lun, Treatise on Damage [due to] Cold),* or some other such hoary classic. *Do not do this!* As a beginner, you should start with something simple and work up to more difficult reading. If you start with something too difficult at the beginning, you will quickly become disheartened and will give up the whole endeavor. Therefore, I cannot stress too highly starting with the appropriate types of literature.

Classical Chinese

Much of the premodern Chinese medical literature is written in *gu wen. Gu* (古) means ancient and *wen* (文) means language or literature. This is also sometimes referred to as *wen yan.* In this case, *wen* means literature and *yan* (言) means speech. So this is not only an ancient form of Chinese, it is a highly stylized, literary language with its own conventions, grammar, and vocabulary. *Even for Chinese* this is a foreign language which must be studied and mastered over many years. It is not something that a Chinese medical student at one of the provincial TCM colleges in China can just pick up and read. You and I cannot pick up *Beowulf* or even Chaucer and read it by sight without notes and commentary. The same is true for the classical Chinese medical literature.[1]

Those of us who have studied Chinese medical pediatrics know that babies' stomachs are immature and inefficient. Therefore, it is important to give babies the right kind of easily digestible food in the right amounts. Otherwise the child may develop food stagnation which may damage the spleen, inhibit the qi, transform heat, and engender dampness and phlegm, thus setting up a series of disease mechanisms which may remain in effect throughout the patient's entire subsequent life. Similarly, if we try to read classical Chinese too early on, it may ruin our "digestion and assimilation" of Chinese for years to come, maybe even our entire life.

Below is a photocopy of a page out of a premodern medical text. It is written in complicated characters, there is no punctuation, and the quality of the printing makes many characters hard to decipher. Do not waste your time with this. Move on to something easier to read. We all think that the old classics are treasure troves of ancient medical secrets. Largely they are not. What has proven valuable and enduring from these classics has mostly been integrated into modern Chinese medicine by previous generations of great Chinese medical scholars. Most of us can profitably spend several years reading the modern Chinese medical literature which will exponentially improve both our theoretical understanding and our clinical practice.

---

[1] "If Confucius could undergo a resurrection he would be quite unable to carry on a conversation with one of his descendants today. Nor would the two be able to communicate in writing unless the present-day descendant of the sage had received a more than average education. Comparable to that of a modern European who has learned to read Latin. Classical written Chinese differs so much from the written language of today that intensive training is needed to master both." John De Francis, *The Chinese Language: Fact and Fantasy, op.cit.,* p. 39

當安徐勿令怖也又天雷勿塞其耳但作餘小聲以亂之也
凡小兒微驚者以長血脉但不欲大驚大驚乃灸驚脉
小兒有熱不欲哺乳臥不安又數驚此癇之初也服紫丸便
愈不差更服之兒立夏後有病治之慎勿妄灸又臍中以膏塗
以除熱湯浴之除熱散赤亦青摩之又臍中以膏塗一
之令兒在涼處勿禁水漿常以新水飲之兒眠時小驚者一
月輒一以紫丸下之減其盛氣令兒不病也
小兒氣盛有病但下之必無所損若不時下則將成病固難
治矣
小兒冬月下無所畏長夏月下難差然有癖者不可不下
凡下四味紫丸最善雖下不損人足以去疾若四味紫丸
熱不盡當按方作龍膽湯稍稍增服之并摩赤膏
不時下者當以赤丸下之赤丸不下當更倍之若已下而餘
後腹中當有小脹滿故當節哺乳數日不可妄下又乳哺小兒
當下之無不差若不下則致寒熱或反吐而發癇或更致下
有小不調也當服紫丸微者少與藥令內消甚者十許日微者五六
而酣者此挾實熱宜下乳令內消甚者少與藥令小
凡小兒屎黃而臭者此腹中有伏熱宜微將服龍膽湯則病易
耗搜而病速愈
增令小下皆須節乳哺數日令胃氣平和若不節乳哺則病易
復令小下之則傷其胃氣令腹脹滿用此下之皆當作癇矣
凡小兒有癖脉大必發癇而不時下致於發癖則難治也若早下
與二指脉不可令起而不時下致於發癖則難治也若早下

之。此脉終不起也脉在掌中尚可早治若至指則病增也
凡小兒腹中有疾生則身寒熱寒熱則血脉動血脉動則心
不定則易驚驚則癇發速也
龍膽湯治小兒出腹血脉盛實寒熱溫壯四肢驚掣發熱
吐唎者若已能進哺中食實不消壯熱及變蒸不解中客人
鬼氣并諸驚癇方悉主之十歲以下小兒皆服之小兒龍膽
湯第一此是出腹嬰兒方若日月長大者以次依此為例若
必知客忤及魅氣者可加人參當歸各如龍膽多少也一百
日兒加半分二百日加一分一歲兒加半兩餘藥皆準爾

龍膽　鉤藤　柴胡去苗　黃芩　桔梗
芍藥　茯神　甘草炙　蜣蜋　大黃

右十味㕮咀以水二升煮取五合為一劑也取之如後
節度藥有虛實虛藥宜足數合水也兒生一日至七日分
一合為三服兒生八日至十五日分一合半為三服兒生
十六日至二十日分二合為三服兒生三十日
分三合為三服兒生三十日至四十日盡以五合為三服
十歲亦準此皆灊下即止勿後服也

治少小心腹熱除熱丹參赤膏方

丹參　雷丸　芒消　戎鹽　大黃各三兩

右伍味切以苦酒半升浸四種一宿以成煉豬脂一斤煎
三上三下去滓內苦消膏成以摩心下冬夏可用一方但

治少小新生肌膚幻弱喜為風邪所中身體壯熱或中大風
手足驚掣五物甘草生摩膏方

甘草炙　防風各一兩　白朮　雷丸半兩　桔梗

右伍味切以不中水豬肪一斤微火煎為膏去滓取彈丸

Qian Jin Yi Fang (Sun Si-miao's Supplementary Formulas to the Thousand [Pieces of] Gold)

The modern Chinese medical literature

As mentioned in the Preface, each year, hundreds of books on all aspects of Chinese medicine are published in China as well as tens of thousands of articles in Chinese TCM journals. Thus there is plenty to read no matter where your particular interest lies: Chinese medicinals, acupuncture, *tui na*, gynecology, pediatrics, geriatrics, or andrology. In general, modern Chinese medical books are roughly divided into basic textbooks (such as on basic Chinese medical theory, acupuncture, Chinese medicinals, or *tui na*), clinical manuals in various specialties, case history collections, and medical essays.

壁赋》与《后赤壁赋》等更是要求背得滚瓜烂熟，一气呵成，当时觉得乏味，却不料古文程度与日俱增，从此博览群书亦觉易也。"所以秦老也希望我们多学文史知识，努力提高文学修养，才能信步漫游于浩如烟海的书林之中。他曾说："专一地研讨医学可以掘出运河，而整个文学修养的提高，则有助于酿成江海。"

名师门下出高徒，与秦老同学者有程门雪、章次公、张赞臣、黄文东等，都成为祖国医学近代史上的耆宿。解放前，人称秦伯未、程门雪、章次公为上海医界三杰。程老精伤寒之学，又推崇叶桂，章老善于本草，自有独到，秦老精于内经，有秦内经之美誉。

秦老又被誉为诗、书、医三绝。他早年即加入柳亚子创立的南社，有"南社题名最少年"句。三十岁时，有《秦伯未诗词集》，四十岁时增订补辑为《谦斋诗词集》七卷，凡三百四十又四首。书法赵之谦，比较工整，蝇头小楷浑匀流丽，非常可爱，行草不多，隶书推崇杨藐翁，现上海城隍庙大殿上的一副对联即他早年墨迹，笔力精神，跃然可见。其实他何止三绝，绘画也颇见功力，善画梅、兰、竹、菊、荷，金石铁笔也十分喜爱，曾有印谱行世。

秦老出师后，即悬壶诊病，同时在中医专门学校执教，一九二四年任江苏中医联合会编辑，后又创办新中医社，主编《中医世界》。一九二八年与杭州王一仁、苏州王慎轩等创办上海中国医学院于上海闸北老靶子路，初期自任教务，倾心治学，勤于著述，工作常无暇日，读书必至更深。教授方

4

Paul Unschuld, the foremost living Western sinologist, has created a two volume set of books on how to learn to read modern medical Chinese. These are titled, *Learn to Read Chinese*. I'll have some good things to say about these books further on. However, Dr. Unschuld (Ph.D.) has based his choice of reading material on his experiences as an academician teaching graduate school sinologists. Therefore, he chose an excellent introductory text on Chinese medical theory by Qin Bo-wei, the 中医入门 (*Zhong Yi Ru Men, An Introduction to Chinese Medicine*) or, more literally, *Entering the Gate of Chinese Medicine*). This text is written as a series of essays, and essays are what I would call "grammar rich and text dense." In other words, these essays are made up of paragraphs which in turn are made up of complete sentences, and these sentences contain grammar. This grammar may be simpler in many ways than typical Indo-European grammar, but there is still grammar nonetheless. By text dense, I mean if you were to look at a page of one of these essays, there would be little white space. Rather, there would be block after block of thick, dense text. Above is an example of a page from a medical essay written by Qin Bo-wei. You could look up every one of the words on this page, but, as a beginner, this is going to take a long, long time.

Clinical manuals

Therefore, I recommend beginning Chinese-to-English translators to begin with modern clinical manuals and formula compendia. (We have already translated some sections from these kinds of books above.) These clinical manuals are written in outline form. Typically, many of the sections are not complete sentences from the English point of view and have little if any grammar. The material is both pithy and succinct (read: not too many words to look up), but the material is immediately clinically useful. As clinicians, every day we are faced with patients who come to us with this or that disease. Our job is to treat those diseases. Therefore, mostly what we as clinicians need to know is how to treat this or that disease.

Below is a page from the kind of clinical manual I suggest beginners work with first. As you will see, it is set up in outline form. There are no dense blocks of text. As we will see in a moment, what we need as clinicians is right there: main signs and symptoms, pattern discrimination, treatment principles, and treatment plans.

（二）证治方法

1. 阴虚火旺

辨证特征　阳强不倒，欲念难除，茎睾胀痛，头晕耳鸣，心烦少寐，腰膝痠软，舌质红少或薄黄、脉弦细数。

治疗方法　滋肾降火。

常用方知柏地黄丸。

2. 肝火内炽

辨证特征　阴茎易举，持久不萎，面红目赤，两胁胀满，急躁易怒，溲黄便干。舌红苔黄，脉弦数。

治疗方法清肝泻火。

常用方　龙胆泻肝汤。

3．败精阻窍

辨证特征　阳强不倒，茎睾胀痛，小便赤涩疼痛频数，少腹拘急，阴囊潮湿、或见尿中白浊。舌质红，苔白中厚腻，脉弦滑。

治疗方法　通精开窍。

常用方　程氏萆薢分清饮。

4．药物劫阴

辨证特征　过用助阳药物后，阳强不倒，时久茎痛，勃起时并无性欲要求，睾丸坠胀，少腹拘急。舌质红，苔白，脉沉弦。

治疗方法　抑阳倒戈。

常用方　黄连猪肚丸。

5．瘀血阻络

辨证特征　外伤后阴茎举而不萎、肿胀疼痛、色紫暗，睾丸时痛，茎睾触之痛甚，舌质紫暗或有瘀斑，苔白，脉沉弦或沉涩。

治疗方法　活血定痛。

常用方　乳香定痛散。

We will look at this page in some detail further on.

Clinical manuals can be purchased at large Chinese bookstores in Chinatowns in North America. In particular, the following Chinese language bookstores have good selections of Chinese medical books and will handle mail or fax orders with a credit card number.

Sino-United Bookstore (LA) Tel. (818)293-3386; Fax (818) 293-3385
Eastwind Books & Arts, Inc. (SF) Tel. (415)772-5888; Fax (415)772-5885
Oriental Cultural Enterprises, Inc. (NY) Tel. (212)226-8461; Fax (212)431-6695
Sino-United Bookstore (Vancouver) Tel. (604)688-3785; Fax (604)688-0798
Sino-United Bookstore (Toronto) Tel. (416)293-2696; Fax (416)293-9716

If you can go to the bookstore yourself, that's the best. Then you can browse through the stacks by yourself. Who knows what you'll come across? In order to find the section of the bookstore where the Chinese medical books are kept, you will need to look for these characters:

中医　　　　　　　*zhong yi*, Chinese medicine

Other characters which can help you identify sections and book contents are listed below:

针灸　　　　　　*zhen jiu*, acupuncture & moxibustion
中药　　　　　　*zhong yao*, Chinese medicinals
草 药　　　　　　*cao yao*, herbal medicine
本草　　　　　　*ben cao*, materia medica

方剂	*fang ji,* formulas & prescriptions
内科	*nei ke,* internal medicine
妇科	*fu ke,* gynecology
儿科	*er ke,* pediatrics
皮肤科	*pi fu ke,* dermatology
眼科	*yan ke,* ophthalmology
耳鼻喉科	*er bi hou ke,* ear, nose, throat
口腔科	*kou qiang ke,* stomatology
正骨科	*zheng gu ke,* orthopedics
伤科	*shang ke,* traumatology
外科	*wai ke,* external medicine
肿瘤科	*zhong liu ke,* tumorology
男科	*nan ke,* andrology
老年科	*lao nian ke,* geriatrics
精神神究科	*jing shen shen jing ke,* psychiatry-neurology
饮食疗法	*yin shi liao fa,* dietary therapy
推拿	*tui na,* Chinese medical massage
气功	*qi gong,* qi gong
医案	*yi an,* case histories
经验	*jing yan,* experiences
中西医结合	*zhong xi yi jie he,* integrated Chinese-Western medicine

Typically, books published in the People's Republic of China are much cheaper than in the U.S. As a beginning translator, I recommend buying a number of smaller, cheaper books and staying away from investing in huge tomes (which you may never be able to read!). Be sure that the book was printed in the PRC as opposed to Hong Kong, Taiwan, or Singapore. Remember, you are looking for books printed with simplified characters. Books which have been printed in the 1990s will often have their bibliographic page (that means the page which tells where and when they were printed) on the back of the title page just like most Western books. However, books printed in the PRC in the 1980s and before typically have this information printed on the bottom of the back cover or the bottom of the last page. I recommend that you only purchase books printed in the 1980s and '90s. These will be up to date and are not likely to contain too much Communist political propaganda.

食 物 中 药 与 便 方

（增订本）

叶桔泉 编著

马永华 叶加南 助编

出 版： 江苏科学技术出版社
发 行： 江苏省 新华 书店
印 刷： 南京人民印刷厂

开本787×1092毫米 1/32 印张12.875 插页 2 字数28万
1973年11月第 1 版 1977年 1 月第 2 版
1980年 9 月第 3 版 1980年 9 月第 1 次印刷
印数 1 —65,000册

书号14196·052 定价0.95元

Above is an example of a typical Chinese bibliographic page. It is from the Chinese dietary therapy book we translated from in the previous chapter. The bold-faced characters in the center of the page are the name of the book. In parentheses under that it says revised and enlarged edition. The next line is the author's name. Under that there are the names of two assistant authors. Then there are three lines of text between two black rules. The first line says the publisher's name. The second line says the distributor's name. And the third line says the name of the printer. Under the second black rule, there are four more lines of text. The first line begins with the term "format" followed by the size of the book in mm. I'm not sure about the two middle numbers (12.875 and 2), but the number of characters in this book seems to be 28 ten thousands or 280,000 characters. The next line down tells us that the first printing occurred in Nov. 1973. The second printing took place Jan. 1977. Line three tells us that the third printing took place Sept. 1980. And I believe the second part of this line tells us that Sept. 1980 was the first printing (of this revised and expanded edition).

Frankly, I'm a little perplexed about the exact meaning of this second part. I've looked up all the words in the dictionary and thought about what they could mean in relationship to all the other words. If I really want to know what these words mean, I will need to find one of my Chinese friends and ask them. In any case, line number four tells us that 65,000 copies of this book were printed. Underneath the third rule, there are two numbers. One seems to be some sort of registration number: Book number 14196.052. The number on the right is the price: 0.95 *yuan*.

A *yuan* is a Chinese "dollar." In 1983, there were, if I remember correctly, 7 *yuan* to a U.S. dollar at official exchange rates and more like 10-12 *yuan* to the dollar on the black market. At black market rates, that means this book cost me $.10 in 1983 when I bought it in China! Today, here in the states, this book is still going to cost you less than $10.

Chinese medical journals

Each province in the People's Republic of China publishes a Chinese medical journal. In addition, many of the TCM colleges and many specialty associations also publish journals. Because of the compact nature of the written Chinese language, each issue of each journal commonly includes 40-50 articles of varying lengths. That means that these journals publish tens of thousands of articles on Chinese medicine per year, virtually none of which are translated in English. The Chinese medical journals contain different types of articles. There are profiles of famous *lao zhong yi,* old Chinese doctors (老中医), there are essays about the teachings of past great masters, there are essays on new uses of ancient formulas, and there are essays on various medical subjects and problems. However, the easiest and some of the most useful information published in these Chinese journals are reports of clinical audits.

Clinical audits are retrospective, non-randomized, non-blinded assessments of the clinical outcomes of various protocols, formulas, or techniques. X number of patients were treated with such and such a treatment and this is what happened. This is what is called "out-come based research." More and more people are realizing that the randomized, double blind, placebo-controlled prospective studies that are currently considered the "gold standard" of scientific research are, in fact, not accurate measures of clinical reality and are way too expensive for what you get. They may be statistically very elegant and they may answer what does exactly what and why, but they are often divorced from the real-life needs of living patients. Clinical audits are statistical assessments of what happened to real-life patients who knowingly chose their own doctors and forms of treatment. This means that clinical audits tell us about people making medical decisions just like you and your patients do.

Typically, these clinical audits are written in outline form. They are not text dense or grammar rich and there is still usually lots of white space on the page. They follow a very *pro forma* outline which is repeated from article to article. Therefore, once one understands the basic categories in one of these articles one can easily access clinically useful information from that article and others like it. Below is a sample one page article from a Chinese TCM journal. Later, we will look at such an article in more detail. Here I only want you to get a sense of how such an article typically looks on a page as opposed to the following page which is a text dense, grammar rich article on The Treatment Method of Using Emotions to Overcome Emotions.

一贯煎治疗经行头痛 148 例

韩风云

（天津市北辰医院）

笔者多年来，用一贯煎为主，加减治疗经行头痛 148 例，取得满意疗效，现报告如下：

1 临床资料

门诊病人 98 例，住院病人 50 例。年龄 15—25 岁，25 例；26—36 岁，38 例；39—49 岁，80 例；50 岁以上 5 例，病程 1—6 月，32 例；7—12 月，40 例；1—3 年，57 例；3—5 年，15 例；5 年以上，4 例。兼痛经者 28 例，兼发热者 12 例，兼呕吐者 37 例，兼情志异常者 13 例，兼经量过少者 34 例，兼经量过多者 24 例。

2 诊断标准

诊断标准，参照 1990 年内蒙古扎兰屯“全国中医第二次脑病会议”所制定的头痛诊断标准，并将此诊断标准应用范围扩大。

3 治疗方法

药物组成：沙参、麦冬、当归、生地、熟地各 20g，川楝子、鳖甲各 10g，枸杞子、阿胶各 20g，白芍 25g，鹿角霜、香附各 15g，加水适量，煎至，150ml，早晚分服；兼痛经进加益母草 30g，木香 12g；兼发热者加地骨皮 15g，丹皮 10g；兼呕吐者加半夏 10g，竹茹 15g，兼情志异常者加酸枣仁 15g，百合 25g；兼经量过多者加升麻　10g，黄芪 30g；兼经量过少者加太子参 20g，川芎 20g。

4 疗效评定标准

疗效评定标准参照 1986 年 6 月南通“第一次全国中医脑病工作会议”制定的疗效判定标准。

1、痊愈：临床症状消失，头痛及主要兼症消除，随访半年未复发。

2、好转：临床症状基本消失，头痛随访三个月未复发。

3、无效：临床症状治疗前后无改变。

5 治疗结果

治疗后不仅经行头痛得以痊愈或好转，其兼症均消失。痊愈 124 例，好转 22 例，无效 2 例。服药后 1—3 剂好转或痊愈者 85 例，4—6 剂好转或痊愈者 61 例，9 剂以上仍头痛 2 例，为无效。

6 典型病例

王某，女，42 岁，三年前恰值月经来潮，头痛加剧，口服“正痛片”、“脑宁”、“镇脑宁”等未效，口出秽语、打人毁物，被送至某院，行电击疗法，离院后遵医嘱长期口服奋乃静 4mgtid，安坦 4mgtid，二年未间断，一年前因故停药一周，又逢月经来临，症见：精神症状如初，头痛难忍，欲吐，经量减少，色淡，心悸，少寐，消瘦，舌淡、边有牡龈，脉细数无力。当拟滋阴养之法，方用一贯益加减。

This is what you want to read.

以情胜情疗法探赜

南京中医药大学 （210029）　**李益生**

关键词　以情胜情疗法　临床应用

以情胜情疗法首载于《内经》，汉代以前即广泛应用，是一种独特的心理疗法。据有的学者统计，现存历代医案中，心理治疗医案有数千例，而大部分都运用了以情胜情疗法，积累了丰富的经验。本文拟对此疗法作一探讨。

《素问·阴阳应象大论》与《素问·五运行大论》均指出：怒伤肝，悲胜怒；喜伤心，恐胜喜；思伤脾，怒胜思；忧伤肺，喜胜忧；恐伤肾，思胜恐。可见以情胜情就是有意识地采用某一种情志活动，去战胜、控制因另一种情志刺激而引起的疾病，从而达到愈病的目的。

以情胜情疗法所依据的基本理论是：人有七情，分属五脏，五脏与情志之间存在着五行制胜的关系。情志活动可以影响人体的阴阳气血，超常的、持久的情志刺激可能引起疾病的发生，而正确地运用情志之偏，则能使机体恢复平衡而病愈。如王冰在注解《素问·五运行大论》时说："怒则不思，忿而忘祸，则胜可知矣。思甚不解，以怒制之，调性之道也。"中医学正是正确地认识到了精神因素与内脏之间及情志与情志之间，在生理病理上存在着相互影响的辩证关系，从而巧妙地运用"以偏救偏"的原理，创立了"以情胜情"的独特疗法。正如吴昆在《医方考·情志门》中所说："情志过极，非药可愈，须以情胜……《内经》一言，百代宗之，是无形之药也。"

情志既可致病，又能治病，这一独到见解深化了医学科学关于情志活动对人体影响的认识。因此，以情胜情疗法一直为中医学家所重视。金元著名医家张从正在《儒门事亲·九气感疾更相为治衍》中说："悲可以治怒，以怆恻苦楚之言感之；喜可以治悲，以谑浪亵狎之言娱之；恐可以治喜，以恐惧死亡之言怖之；怒可以治思，以污辱欺罔之言触之；思可以治恐，以虑彼忘此之言夺之。""余又尝以巫跃妓抵以治人之悲结者；余又尝以针下之时便杂舞，忽笛鼓应之，以治人之忧而心痛者；余尝拍击门窗，使其声不绝，以治因惊而畏响，魂气飞扬者；余又尝治一妇人久思

而不眠，余假醉而不问，妇果呵怒，是夜困睡。"张氏的医疗活动，使以情胜情疗法从理论到实践均得到了深化和发展。当然，运用以情胜情疗法，不能简单地按五行制胜的模式机械照搬，而应以病理生理的实际作为基础，灵活而巧妙地进行设计、应用。

从历代运用以情胜情疗法案例及本人的体会来看，多数是通过激发某种情志活动来治疗情志病变及由情志变动过度所引起的躯体病变。具体可归纳为以下四种方法。

1　激怒疗法

愤怒本属一种不良情绪，然而愤怒又为阳性情绪活动，适当地激发愤怒，可以起到忘却思虑、排遣忧愁、消散郁结、抑制惊喜的作用，并能促使阳气升发、气机运动，营血周流。故恰当利用激怒的心理疗法，常可治疗因思虑过度而气结、忧愁不解而意志消沉、惊恐太过而胆虚气怯等阴性情志病变。

运用激怒疗法必须注意分寸，要以将消极因素转化为积极因素为目的。如莫枚士《研经言·五志论》所说："故肝为怒，怒生于恨，成于愤。恨而不已，为怨，为愠，为恚；愤而不已，为奋，为发、为自强。"笔者经临床实践体会到，本法的操作在于通过言语交谈激发病人的自尊和自信，进而以疏导解除其情志症结，可采用对比、激励等手段进行。如治一张姓女青年，高中毕业分配到幼儿园当保育员，感到自己地位低下，前途渺茫，经常称病在家，渐渐发展到不思茶饭、卧床不起，或面壁独坐，神志萎靡，寡言少语，精神病院诊为抑郁症。来诊时蓬头垢面，衣衫不整，意志消沉。笔者向家属详询病史后，首先从女青年应有的基本修养谈起，针对其装束举止进行严厉指责批评，使其自尊心受到很大触动。接着又列举一些青年在平凡工作中做出不平凡贡献的事实，激发其自信心和事业心，并配用逍遥散和越鞠丸疏肝理气解郁。经多次心理、药物治疗，病人精神状态有了很大改善，逐步愉快地投入到工作中去。此例

533

This is what you want to stay away from as a beginner.

The good news is that you can order any of the Chinese TCM journals by mail. Write to:

China International Book Trading Corporation
P.O. Box 399, Beijing, PRC

Ask them to send you their latest catalog and price list of Chinese periodicals. This will be a newspaper like affair with hundreds of names of Chinese periodicals. Your job is to find the ones on Chinese medicine. Below is a photocopy of part of the TCM section from the 1998 catalog.

Code	Title	Publisher			
0140M	中医杂志 * *	中国中医药学会、中国中医研究院	23.16	18.10	35.50
0141M	上海中医药杂志 *	上海中医学院、上海中医学会	23.16	18.10	36.90
0185M	浙江中医杂志 *	浙江省中医研究院	17.40	18.10	35.50
0186M	新中医 *	广州中医药大学	20.28	18.10	39.80
0299BM	中国医学文摘——中医 *	中国中医研究院中医药信息研究所	13.86	9.10	19.90
0326BM	云南中医中药杂志 * *	云南省中医中药研究所	10.14	9.10	19.20
0342BM	浙江中医学院学报 * *	浙江中医学院	8.70	9.10	23.50
0354BM	中医教育 *	北京中医药大学	7.20	9.10	17.80
0518BM	山东中医药大学学报 *	山东中医药大学	8.70	9.10	21.40
0530M	辽宁中医杂志 * *	辽宁中医学院、辽宁省中医药学会	17.40	9.90	24.30
0618BM	福建中医药 *	福建省中医药学会、福建中医学院	5.76	9.10	18.50
0640M	中国中西医结合杂志 * *	中国中西医结合学会中国中医研究院	28.32	18.10	41.20
0668BM	北京中医 *	北京中医药学会	13.02	9.10	19.90
0671M	陕西中医 *	中国中医药学会陕西分会	17.40	18.10	36.90
0695BM	河南中医 *	河南中医学院、河南省中医药学会	8.70	9.10	19.90
0734BM	北京中医药大学学报 * *	北京中医药大学	8.70	9.10	19.90
0753BM	湖北中医杂志 *	湖北中医学院	7.20	9.10	19.20
0823M	四川中医	四川省中医学会	14.40	18.10	36.90
0826M	山东中医杂志 *	山东中医药学会、山东中医药大学	11.52	9.90	22.90
0846BM	吉林中医药 *	长春中医学院	5.76	5.00	12.20
0952Q	甘肃中医学院学报 *	甘肃中医学院	3.84	6.10	13.30
0968BM	中国医药学报 * *	中国中医药学会	13.86	9.10	20.60
0977BM	山西中医 *	山西省中医药学会	8.70	9.10	18.50
1011M	江苏中医 *	江苏省卫生厅	23.16	18.10	49.90
1012BM	江西中医药 *	江西中医药学会、江西中医学院	5.22	9.10	19.90
1040BM	天津中医 *	天津中医学院	10.14	9.10	18.50
1102BM	湖南中医杂志 *	湖南省中医药研究院	11.58	9.10	22.10
1111BM	中医研究 * *	河南省中医药研究院	7.50	9.10	19.20
1125BM	中医药学报 *	黑龙江中医学院	6.36	9.10	19.20
1142SM	实用中西医结合杂志 * *	中国中西医结合学会	46.08	36.20	82.50
1157BM	黑龙江中医药 * *	黑龙江省中医研究院	5.76	9.10	19.20
1163BM	中医函授通讯 * *	辽宁中医学院	11.40	9.10	18.50
1172BM	中医药信息 *	黑龙江中医学院	5.76	9.10	19.20
1266BM	中国中医急症 * *	国家中医药管理局医政司	5.76	5.00	12.20
1271Q	天津中医学院学报 *	天津中医学院	3.84	6.10	11.40
1296BM	中国中医骨伤科 * *	中国中医药学会、湖北省中医药研究	12.12	9.10	19.20
1310M	中华医学杂志(英文版) * *	中华医学会	144.60	18.10	49.90
4333Q	陕西中医学院学报 *	陕西中医学院	2.88	6.10	11.90
4334BM	陕西中医函授	陕西中医学院	3.48	9.10	17.80
4417BM	国医论坛 *	南阳中医学校	7.20	9.10	17.80
4418Q	中西医结合肝病杂志 * *	湖北中医学院	7.72	6.10	12.80
4431BM	甘肃中医 *	甘肃省卫生厅	5.76	5.00	12.20
4470BM	光明中医 *	中国民间中医药协会	9.24	9.10	19.20
4471Q	福建中医学院学报 * *	福建中医学院	3.84	6.10	12.30
4506BM	实用中医药杂志 * *	重庆市中医管理局	8.70	9.10	17.80
4690M	中国中医基础医学杂志 * * ☆	中国中医研究院基础所	32.40	18.10	42.70
6062Q	湖南中医学院学报 * ☆	湖南中医学院	5.80	6.10	14.70
6080Q	河南医科大学学报 * ☆	河南医科大学	9.64	10.80	24.30
0491M	气 功 *	浙江省中医药研究院	9.24	9.90	20.00
0497M	中国针灸 * *	中国针灸学会	34.68	18.10	38.40
0654M	气功与科学	广东省气功科学研究协会	18.48	18.10	36.90
0657BM	上海针灸杂志 * *	上海市针灸学会、上海中医药研究院	11.58	9.10	23.50
0702BM	中华气功	中国中医药学会	24.84	5.00	12.20
0970M	气功与体育 *	陕西省新闻出版局	16.20	18.10	35.50
1034M	中国气功	河北省北戴河气功康复医院	16.20	9.90	24.30
1088M	针灸临床杂志 * *	黑龙江中医药大学	17.40	18.10	38.40
1130BM	东方气功	北京气功研究会	9.24	9.10	17.80
4605BM	中医外治杂志 *	山西省中医药学会	7.20	5.00	10.70
0221M	中草药 * *	国家医药管理局中草药情报中心站	104.04	18.10	41.20
0399M	中国中药杂志 * *	中国药学会	43.56	18.10	41.20
1093M	中成药 * *	国家医药管理局中成药信息中心	43.56	18.10	38.40

These are the journals having to do with Chinese medicine. On the left is the order number. Then comes the journal title. Then comes the work unit which publishes the journal. Then come a series of numbers. These numbers are U.S. $. The first number is the unit price. The second number is the yearly subscription price. The third number is the *additional* surface postage (takes six weeks to three months, but who cares?). And the fourth number is the *additional* airmail postage.

First pick the journals you want. The following ones are all good choices as far as I'm concerned.

北京中医	*Bei Jing Zhong Yi, Beijing Chinese Medicine*
上海中医杂志	*Shang Hai Zhong Yi Yao Za Zhi, Shanghai Journal of Chinese Medicine & Medicinals*
新中医	*Xin Zhong Yi, New Chinese Medicine*
浙江中医杂志	*Zhe Jiang Zhong Yi Za Zhi, Zhejiang Journal of Chinese Medicine*
四川中医	*Si Chuan Zhong Yi, Sichuan Chinese Medicine*
中国针灸	*Zhong Guo Zhen Jiu, Chinese Acupuncture & Moxibustion*

When you look at the China International Book Trading Corporation catalog, you may see the titles of a number of potentially very interesting journals. You can find journals of orthopedics, journals of infertility, journals of ophthalmology. However, if these journals do not have the words 中医 (*zhong yi*, Chinese medicine) in their title, they are probably Western medical journals. If you order one of these thinking that you are going to get a journal specializing in a certain area of Chinese medicine, you are going to be disappointed. Not only will there be little if anything about the specialty and Chinese medicine, the vocabulary will all be a technical Western medical vocabulary which will be very difficult to translate.

Likewise, the 中西医结合杂志 (*Zhong Xi Yi Jie He Za Zhi, Journal of Integrated Chinese-Western Medicine*) may appear, at first sight, a very useful to journal to which to subscribe. Certainly it does contain some very interesting and useful information. However, its articles tend to be written by Western MD's with an interest in Chinese medicine rather than by practitioners of primarily Chinese medicine, and, therefore, the style and terminology is very much Western medicine. That makes most of the articles published in this journal hard to read, and not always very useful for the non-MD practitioner of Chinese medicine. Very often the treatments described in this journal fall outside our legal scope of non-MD acupuncturists' practice in the West.

My suggestion is to pick a couple of expensive TCM journals and then pick a few cheaper ones. This should give you a good selection of what's being published around China today. For two hundred dollars U.S., you can have more Chinese TCM journals pouring into your office every month than you will know what to do with. But you will be building a very useful clinical library for when your reading Chinese begins to pick up speed.

10
The Art of Interpretation

Basically, what I am advocating is dictionary translation. When presented with a page from a Chinese clinical manual or Chinese TCM journal, you simply look up every word, word by word. Then you try to string these meanings together to make some coherent sense. *There are two reasons why this is actually possible.* The first is that the Chinese language does not use much in the way of grammar the way we are used to thinking of and learning grammar.[1] The language is much looser and open-ended than English which is so linear and precise. Chinese is more relational or positional and leaves a lot to interpretation.

Secondly, you already know something about the material you are trying to read. My assumption is that you are either a student at a Western acupuncture/Chinese medical school or are a professional practitioner of acupuncture and Chinese medicine. In either case, you do already know a lot about the material you are trying to read. When it comes to picking whether, in a given context, a Chinese character means this or that of its possible dictionary definitions, you should have an easier time because you already know something about the context. However, before we immediately dive in trying to translate something, we need to know just a little bit about Chinese word order, compound terms, and other "grammatical" issues.

Compound terms

Every individual character in Chinese is a word in and of itself. However, complex concepts are typically made up of two or more characters. When two characters are combined to form a single concept, this is called a compound term. Below are some examples of compound terms where the combination of two characters modifies the meaning of either one or both of those characters.

中(*zhong*, middle or China/Chinese) + 医 (*yi*, medicine or doctor) = 中医, *zhong yi*, Chinese medicine or a Chinese doctor

西 (*xi*, West or Western) + 医 (*yi*, medicine) = 西医 , *xi yi*, Western medicine or a Western MD

医 (*yi*, medicine) + 药 (*yao*, medicinals) = 医药 , *yi yao*, medicinals

草 (*cao*, herbs) + 药(*yao*, medicinals) = 草药 , *cao yao*, herbal medicinals

中(*zhong*, middle or China/Chinese) + 药 (*yao*, medicinal) = 中药 , *zhong yao*, Chinese medicinals

中(*zhong*, middle or China/Chinese) + 草 (*cao*, herbs) + 药 (*yao*, medicinals) = 中草药 , *zhong cao yao*, Chinese herbal medicinals

工 ((*gong*, work) + 人(*ren*, person) = 工人 , *gong ren*, worker

---

[1] I am not really saying that Chinese has *no* grammar. Y.R. Chao's 1968 monumental book, *Grammar of Spoken Chinese*, is more than 800 pages in length. It is that Chinese grammar is very different from English grammar.

药 (*yao*, medicine) + 工 (*gong*, work) + 人 (*ren*, person) = 药工人, *yao gong ren*, medicinal worker

人 (*ren*, person) + 工 (*gong*, work) = 人工, *ren gong*, man-made, *i.e.*, artificial

不 (*bu*, no, not) + 同 (*tong*, same) = 不同, *bu tong*, not the same, *i.e.*, different

不 (*bu*, no, not) + 一 (*yi*, one) = 不一, *bu yi*, not one, *i.e.*, different, not identical

不 (*bu*, no, not) + 可 (*ke*, ok) = 不可, *bu ke*, not ok

不 (*bu*, no, not) + 能 (*neng*, able) = 不能, *bu neng*, not able, cannot, or inability

If you have already studied Western medical terminology, you should already have some feel for how two words can be put together to create a compound term or new concept. In English, our technical medical vocabulary is mostly derived from Greek and Latin. When you studied Western medical terminology, you probably had to learn a certain number of Latin or Greek root words, some prefixes, and some suffixes. The word physiology is made up of two parts. "Physio-" has something to do with the workings of the body, while "-ology" means the study of something. When we put these two together, we create a new word meaning "the study or science of the workings of the body". Appendicitis is made up of the prefix "a", the root "pend", and the suffix "-itis." "Pend" means something that hangs down. "A" means from. So the appendix is something that hangs down from something else. The suffix "-itis" means inflammation. Put them all together and you get inflammation of the thing that hangs down, *i.e.*, the appendix.

Reading the Chinese language is pretty much like taking apart the above Western medical terms. The Chinese frequently like to use two words together. So when you see two words together, you need to think about the individual meanings of each word and then about what they might mean when put together. This takes both left and right sides of the brain or, in other words, both logic *and* intuition. The more you have of both and the more you love language for language's sake, the easier and more enjoyable this process will be. If you are a curious and interested person who likes to solve puzzles, this should actually be a very entertaining and enjoyable process.

Parts of speech

In English, parts of speech, *i.e.*, whether a word is a noun, adjective, verb, adverb, preposition, or conjunction, are typically well defined and often end in certain inflections. Chinese is an uninflected language without declensions or conjugations, and commonly a word can act as either an adjective or noun or even as a noun or a verb without any modification of the word itself. For instance, the word 针 (*zhen*, needle or acupuncture) can also be used as a verb, as in "to needle." Likewise, 灸 (*jiu*, moxibustion) can also be used as verb, as in "to moxa." 上 (*shang*) can be used as either a verb, adverb, noun, adjective, or "preposition." For instance, an inner internal branch of the liver channel *ascends* (verb) to the vertex. The spleen channel runs *upward* (adverb) to the abdomen. 上脘 (*Shang Wan*), Upper (adjective) Stomach Duct, *i.e.*, the name of CV 13. 山上 (*shan shang*) means *on* ("preposition" but actually a postposition) the mountain. Points below may be used to treat *above* (noun). In each of the above four sentences, the italicized word in English is simply 上 (*shang*) in Chinese.

William McNaughton has this to say about Chinese characters and English parts of speech:

> You should try to keep in mind that a Chinese character is not what we think of as a word in English, and that Chinese words for which the characters stand are often subject to different kinds of syntactic restriction. In fact, what we consider nouns, verbs, adjectives, and adverbs in English are, in classical Chinese, all considered one part of speech—any noun can be a verb, adjective, or adverb.[2]

Frequently, the part of speech a character plays in a sentence depends on what other words it is combined with. For instance, 电 (*dian*) means electricity, a noun, all by itself. But it becomes an adjective when it precedes the word 针(*zhen,* needle). Now it means electroacupuncture. 男 (*nan*) means man. As such, it is a noun. When combined with the word 性(*xing,* nature, quality, disposition), it becomes the adjective male. Similarly, 女 (*nu*) means woman, a noun. When it combines with 性, it becomes the adjective female.

Word order

Sometimes in Chinese, the word order is the same as in English. For instance, the verb typically precedes its object: 开门(*kai men,* open the door), 关门 (*guan men,* shut the door), and 上山 (*shang shan,* ascend the mountain).[3] However, what in English are prepositions (literally meaning positioned in front of or before) are commonly in Chinese postpositions (positioned after or behind). Therefore, 山上 (*shan shang*) means *on* the mountain. This word order is just the opposite of English.

Singular & plural

In English, we inflect our nouns to denote number. There is one car but two car*s*. Or we change the form of the noun altogether. There is one man but two men. In Chinese, there are no inflections or changes in writing to denote number, one or more than one. Thus all Chinese nouns are what linguists call mass nouns like the English word deer. They can mean either one or more than one. How then do Chinese know whether the writer is talking about one or more than one whatevers? Simple, by specifying either the exact number or using a second word denoting more than one. So 一人(*yi ren*) is one man, 二人 (*er ren*) is two men, 两人(*liang ren*) is both men, 数人(*shu ren*) is several or many men, and 诸人(*zhu ren*) means all men or various men.

Some common kinds of sentences

There are a few very simple kinds of verbs which are helpful to know when getting started trying to read Chinese. First is the simple stative sentence. In a stative sentence, the main verb or predicate of the sentence is a comment on the nature, status, or condition of the sentence's

---

[2] McNaughton, *op. cit.*, p. 14-15

[3] Therefore, Chinese is described as an SVO language—subject, verb, object.

subject. The subject of the sentence takes no action. In this case, the verb used in this structure is "to be" plus an adjective. In actual fact, the words "to be" do not appear in the Chinese. In this kind of sentence, however, there must be an adverb preceding the adjective. For instance, take the following sentence.

脾不虚 (*Pi bu xu.*) The spleen is/was not vacuous.

In this sentence, the spleen (脾, *pi*) is the noun/subject, the verb "to be" is implicit, the adverb is the word (不, *bu*) or "not", and (虚, *xu*) "vacuous" is the adjective. Here are other examples of this stative construction.

肝阳很旺 (*Gan yang hen wang.*) Liver yang is/was very exuberant.

肾气不固 (*Shen qi bu gu.*) The kidney qi is not/was not secure.

Equative sentences indicate whether or not two things are equal. This type of sentence always uses the verb 是(*shi*, to be). Here, the verb to be does appear in the sentence in Chinese.

她是老中医(*Ta shi lao zhong yi.*) She is an old Chinese doctor.

我是学生 (*Wo shi xue sheng.*) I am a student.

脾是阴脏 (*Pi shi yin zang.*) The spleen is a yin viscus.

Simple functive sentences use verbs to show the actions of their subjects. A simple functive sentence typically consists of three main parts: a subject, the functive verb, and the object.

气行血 (*Qi xing xue.*) The qi moves the blood.

肺主气(*Fei zhu qi.*) The lungs rule the qi.

肝主筋 (*Gan zhu jin.*) The liver governs the sinews.

肾恶寒 (*Shen e han.*) The kidneys are averse to cold.

Simple functive sentences are very common in the Chinese medical literature.

Note in the above examples how I have had to add various English particles to make the sentences sound correct: "*the* kidneys", "*a* yin viscus", "*an* old Chinese doctor." Compared to English, Chinese is very compact, very stripped down, and we often have to add numerous small English words—particles, prepositions, conjunctions, verb forms, single and plural—to make the sentence sound like a native English speaker's.

Doubling up

There are a number of Chinese expressions made by repeating the same word twice. Here are some common ones:

人人　　*ren ren*, people-people, *i.e.*, everybody
天天　　*tian tian*, heaven-heaven or day-day, *i.e.*, every day, daily, day by day
年年　　*nian nian*, year-year, *i.e.*, every year, yearly, year by year
大大　　*da da*, great-great, *i.e.*, very big or greatly
明明　　*ming ming*, clear-clear or bright-bright, *i.e.*, clearly, obviously
连连　　*lian lian*, again-again, *i.e.*, in rapid succession
往往　　*wang wang*, go-go, *i.e.*, often
足足　　*zu zu*, foot-foot, *i.e.*, fully
草草　　*cao cao*, grass-grass, *i.e.*, carelessly, hastily
万万　　*wan wan*, 10,000-10,000, *i.e.*, absolutely, wholly
元元　　*yuan yuan*, source-source or fountainhead-fountainhead, *i.e.*, continuously
略略　　*lue lue*, slight-slight, *i.e.*, very slightly
早早　　*zao zao*, early-early, *i.e.*, very early
少少　　*shao shao*, little bit-little bit, *i.e.*, a very little bit

As you can see from above, sometimes when two words are repeated, they create a completely new concept. Other times, it simply means very much of whatever the word is.

Combining opposites

Frequently, Chinese combines opposites in order to create a new compound term. For instance:

大小　　*Da xiao*, big-small, *i.e.*, size
左右　　*Zuo you*, left-right, *i.e.,* approximately
快慢　　*Kuai man*, fast-slow, *i.e.*, speed
多少　　*Duo shao*, many-few, *i.e.*, amount

Punctuation

Before the influence of Western culture, Chinese was written from top to bottom, right to left, and without punctuation of any kind. In fact, beginning Chinese readers had to spend their first year(s) trying to learn how to group words into their proper sentences. The good news for us is that modern Chinese have adopted basically English punctuation to make things easier as part of their language reform. Chinese books now read horizontally from left to right, and things like commas, colons, periods, parentheses, brackets, and question marks are the norm. However, the English reader should take these with a grain of salt. Chinese often put periods after incomplete sentences and string long groups of sentences together as if they were phrases separated by commas. As we will see below, I do not think we need to slavishly follow Chinese punctuation. I personally do not think Chinese understand English punctuation all that well. It is not even clear to me whether English concepts such as complete and incomplete sentences actually exist in Chinese, since our notion of parts of speech does not exist in Chinese.

Getting started

Find something that you would like to translate, assuming that it is not too text dense and that it is written in modern Chinese with simplified characters. Make a photocopy of the page or paragraph, blowing the characters up so that they are easier to see. Then cut out the characters and paste them onto a piece of paper, being sure to keep them in their correct order. As an alternative to this step, you can try to write out the characters with large strokes with plenty of space underneath each line of characters. However, if you do not write the characters correctly, this will make it even more difficult to look them up. So unless your Chinese penmanship is good, use the photocopier.

Below is an example of how I taught myself to translate and how I encourage my students to begin. First you look up each word in a sentence individually. Under each entry in the dictionary, you are likely to find that there is more than one meaning for any character. If it is immediately obvious which of these meanings fits the present situation, write that down under the character. You might also write down the Pinyin spelling of the character and the tone mark so you can look up the character again quickly if you have to. If you find that the word has several possible definitions, write all of these down under the Chinese character. Then do the same thing for the next character, and the one after that, and so on and so on. You will probably end up with something that looks like the following.

性	早	熟	的	病	因	多	因	疾	病	或	误	服	某
xìng	zǎo	shú	de	bìng	yīn	duō	yīn	jí	bìng	huò	wù	fú	mǒu

些	药	物	本	病	的	病	变	主	要	在	肾	肝
xiē	yào	wù.	běn	bìng	de	bìng	biàn	zhǔ	yào	zài	shèn,	gān

两	脏	其	发	生	多	由	肝	郁	化	火	或	阴
liǎng	zàng,	qí	fā	shēng	duō	yóu	gān	yù	huà	huǒ	huò	yīn

虚	火	旺	相	火	妄	动	所	致
xū	huǒ	wàng,	xiàng	huǒ	wàng	dòng	suǒ	zhì

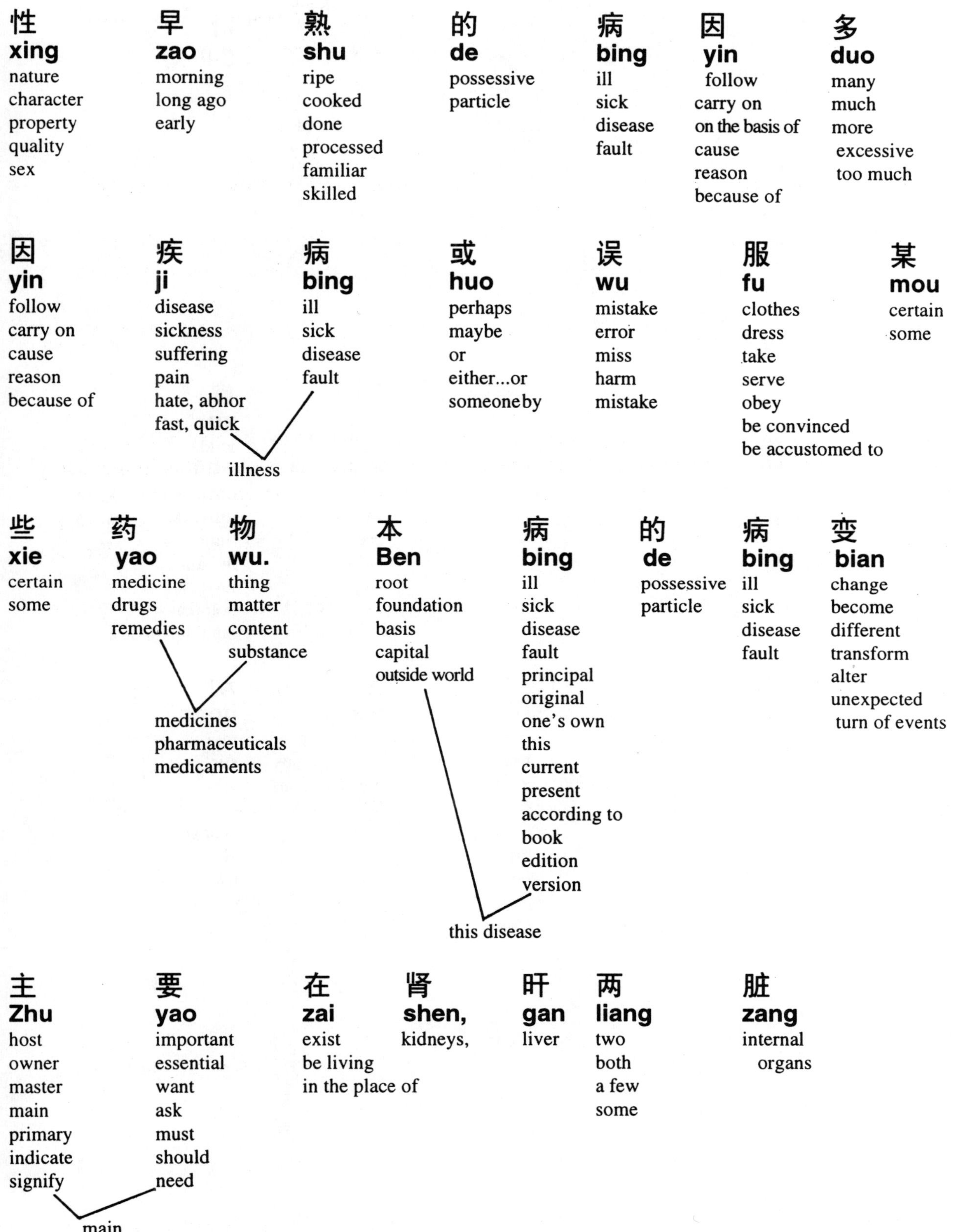

性
xing
nature
character
property
quality
sex

早
zao
morning
long ago
early

熟
shu
ripe
cooked
done
processed
familiar
skilled

的
de
possessive
particle

病
bing
ill
sick
disease
fault

因
yin
follow
carry on
on the basis of
cause
reason
because of

多
duo
many
much
more
excessive
too much

因
yin
follow
carry on
cause
reason
because of

疾
ji
disease
sickness
suffering
pain
hate, abhor
fast, quick

病
bing
ill
sick
disease
fault

或
huo
perhaps
maybe
or
either...or
someone by

误
wu
mistake
error
miss
harm
mistake

服
fu
clothes
dress
take
serve
obey
be convinced
be accustomed to

某
mou
certain
some

illness

些
xie
certain
some

药
yao
medicine
drugs
remedies

物
wu.
thing
matter
content
substance

本
Ben
root
foundation
basis
capital
outside world

病
bing
ill
sick
disease
fault
principal
original
one's own
this
current
present
according to
book
edition
version

的
de
possessive
particle

病
bing
ill
sick
disease
fault

变
bian
change
become
different
transform
alter
unexpected
turn of events

medicines
pharmaceuticals
medicaments

this disease

主
Zhu
host
owner
master
main
primary
indicate
signify

要
yao
important
essential
want
ask
must
should
need

在
zai
exist
be living
in the place of

肾
shen,
kidneys,

肝
gan
liver

两
liang
two
both
a few
some

脏
zang
internal
organs

main

其
qi
his
her
its
their
possessive
pronoun

发
fa
send out
issue
deliver
discharge
shoot
emit
develop
expand

生
sheng
give birth
bear
grow
living
livelihood
unripe
green
unfamiliar
pupil, student
unprocessed

happen, take place

多
duo
many
much
more
excessive
too much

由
you
cause
reason
because of
due to
follow
obey

肝
gan
liver

郁
yu
strongly fragrant
luxurient
lush
gloomy
depressed
sad

化
hua
change
transform
convert
influence
digest
burn up

火
huo
fire
firearms
ammunition
fiery
flaming
urgent
pressing
anger
temper

或
huo
perhaps
maybe
or
either...or
someone

阴
yin
yin
moon
north
shade
back
hidden
negative

虚
xu
void
emptiness
unoccupied
diffident
timid
in vain
false
nominal
humble, modest

火
huo
fire
firearms
ammunition
fiery
flaming
urgent
pressing
anger
temper

旺
wang,
prosperous
flourishing
vigorous

相
xiang
looks
appearance
bearing
posture
assist
prime minister

火
huo
fire
firearms
ammunition
fiery
flaming
urgent
pressing
anger
temper

妄
wang
absurd
preprosterous
presumptuous
rash

动
dong
move
stir
act
get moving
change
alter
use
touch

所
guo
place

致
zhi
send
deliver
extend
devote
incur
result in
cause
manner, style
fine, delicate

be caused by
be the result of

The first three words, *xing zao shu,* are a compound term meaning "premature sexual development". As a compound term, these words need to be looked up in a Chinese-English medical distionary. *De* is a possessive particle. It is followed by *bing yin. Bing* means disease, yin means cause. As a compound term, these two mean "disease cause or etiology". So the first five characters read, "The disease causes of premature sexual development..." *Duo* means "many", "mostly", or "often". Then we have *yin* again, "because", "are due to". This is followed by *ji* which means "disease" and *bing* which means "disease". *Ji bing* as a compound term means "disease". The next character, *huo*, means "maybe, perhaps", or simply "or", as it does here. It is followed by *wu*, "mistake", *fu*, "take or administer", *mou xie*, as compound term for "some", *yao*, "medicine", *wu*, "substances". If we put this all together, the sentence reads: "The disease causes of premature sexual development are mostly due to disease or mistaken administration of some medicines."

Ben means "this". *Bing* means "disease". *De*, is once again a possessive particle. It is followed by *bing*, "disease", *bian*, "changes", *i.e.*, "This disease's pathological changes..." Next we have the coumpound term *zhu yao*, "mainly". *Zai* means "located in", while *shen* means "kidneys". *Gan* means "liver", *liang* means "two", and *zang* means "viscera". Ergo: "This disease's pathological changes mainly reside in the two viscera of the kidneys and liver." The Chinese run this sentence on. We can put a period here to make the thought complete and the English sound OK.

Qi is an all purpose possessive pronoun. It means "his, her, their, its". *Fu sheng* is a compound term meaning "takes place or occurs". Therefore, "Its occurrence..." *Duo* again means "many, mostly, or often". *You* means "because of". "It's occurrence is mostly due to..." *Gan* means "liver", while *yu* means "depression". Now we're in the realm of Chinese medical theory and jargon; so now we need to be looking these Chinese medical technical terms up in Wiseman. *Gan yu* means "liver depression". *Hua* means to "transform". *Huo* means "fire". "It's occurrence is mostly due to liver depression transforming fire..." *Huo* means "or". *Yin* means "yin", *xu* means "vacuity". *Huo* means "fire", and Wiseman translates *wang* as "effulgence". "It's occurrence is mostly due to liver depression transforming fire or yin vacuity fire effulgence,..." *Xiang* means "minister", huo means "fire", *wang* Wiseman translates as "frenetic", and *dong* he translates as "stirring". *Guo zhi* is a compound term meaning "because of". Hence, the whole sentence reads: "It's occurrence is mostly due to liver depression transforming fire, yin vacuity fire effulgence, and ministerial fire stirring frenetically." We can forget the *suo zhi* at the end. We already have our "because of" or "due to".

As you can see from the above example, although each word may have more than a single meaning, in a Chinese medical text, only certain of these meanings will apply. Further, the words in the first part of the sentence will help define how the words in the latter half of the sentence will be used. Therefore, you need to determine the meaning of each word or compound *in context.*

It is important to remember that, although a given Chinese word may have more than a single usage, and, therefore, more than a single definition in English, it is only one word *in Chinese.* Thus it is useful to try to think about how a single concept could encompass all of these definitions.

Let's take the word 活 (*huo*) as an example. This verb often shows up in the compound term (活血, *huo xue*). If we look this word up in a regular Chinese-English dictionary, we will find that it means 1) to live, 2) to be alive, 3) to save, 4) something lively or vivid, or 5) movable or moving. The compound term, *huo xue*, is often translated as activate the blood. However, Nigel Wiseman suggests the term, "to quicken the blood." The word quick in English means something that is lively, moving, and also alive. And if we quicken the dead, that means to save a person's life. In other words, there is a common thread, a single underlying reality which informs and determines all the usages of a single word. As a translator, you want to try to grasp the underlying logic of all the English language definitions for a word given in your Chinese-English dictionary. Then, apparent contradictions or peculiar constructions will begin to come into focus and make more sense.

11
Terminology

When trying to translate Chinese medical texts, we are working on technical non-fiction. The information we are translating is basically instructions to do certain things to real-life people. Therefore, it is extremely important that we translate these instructions correctly and as close to how the author intended as possible. Because this is a technical translation, there is, as in all professions, a technical language or lingo. In the West, the technical language of medicine is made up from Latin and Greek words. These are words which the native English-speaking lay person may be completely ignorant of the meaning. For instance, splenohepatomegaly may be completely meaningless to someone who A) has never studied Greek and B) has never studied Western medicine.

Chinese is different from English in that it is not a language made up from loan words from many other languages. Therefore, the technical jargon of Chinese medicine is mainly made up from everyday Chinese words. However, when used in a technical sense, they take on a technical meaning which may also be opaque to the native Chinese-speaking layperson. In the beginning, Western sinologists thought of Chinese medicine as folk medicine, and, therefore, they failed to appreciate the precision of its technical language. Unfortunately, many of the linguistic conventions we use today when translating this technical literature were erroneously created by people working under this delusion. These early translators either did not bother to translate the technical precision of the Chinese, glossing over it entirely, or wrongly adopted Western medical and biological concepts to stand in for Chinese ones they did not fully comprehend in their Chinese medical sense. For instance, many students tell me they never heard of the concept of counterflow (*ni*, 逆) before studying with me. Their teachers never used this concept. While the concept of sedation is a 180° wrong translation based on misunderstanding the actual Chinese concepts with their full technical implications.

As Nigel Wiseman has pointed out, the word "sedate" comes from the Latin word *sedere*. It means "to sit down and stay put". The Chinese technical term 泻 (*xie*, to drain) means to drain off something that is clogging or obstructing the flow of qi, blood, or body fluids. We definitely do not want to "sedate" such evil repletions. What we want to do is drain and discharge them. To sedate them means to make what is already misplaced, stuck, and obstructing stay where it is all the more firmly.

It was the German sinologist, Manfred Porkert, in the late 1970's who first realized that, when it comes to translating Chinese medicine, we are dealing with a very precise, technical language. Unfortunately, Porkert, being an old school European, chose to use Latin for the creation of a standard, philologically accurate technical translational terminology. He assumed that all educated professionals know at least rudimentary Latin. Sadly, that is no longer the case, and especially so in the United States. Therefore, Porkert's great insight and contribution to the Western study of Chinese medicine has largely been ignored. He took one foreign language and turned it into an equally foreign language!

It was Nigel Wiseman, who, beginning more than 10 years or more ago, set out to create a philologically accurate, technically precise, self-consistent set of English language Chinese medical equivalents. In 1990, Wiseman *et al.* published a *Glossary of Chinese Medical Terms and Acupuncture Points*. This was meant to be a freely available (but not necessarily for free), standard Chinese medical glossary with Chinese characters, Pinyin romanization with tone marks, and suggested standard English translation. Wiseman correctly saw that there are subtle differences in technical meaning between many words used in the Chinese medical literature which previous translators had been glossing over. Therefore, he sought, as far as is possible, to translate one Chinese word with one English word. Using this approach, one should always be able to A) know, by looking up in the glossary, the original Chinese character in question, and B) catch the full technical implications of the Chinese original.

Unfortunately, Wiseman suggested some unusual translations for words which Western students and practitioners had become habituated to — for instance, vacuity instead of deficiency for 虚 (*xu*), repletion instead of excess for 实 (*shi*), drain instead of sedate for 泻 (*xie*), and supplement instead of tonify for 补 (*bu*). Until now, Wiseman's terminology has largely lain unused and even scoffed at because of his choice for these four words. Certainly, they do sound unusual. However, that is exactly part of Wiseman's key point. Technical language conveys special information and may sound strange to the layperson not schooled in this technical language's meaning and use.

Personally, I have found Nigel Wiseman's glossary to be a god-send. The more I learn about the Chinese language, the more I agree with his choices of English language equivalents. I don't have the time or the inclination to devote my life to finding the best English language translation for a Chinese medical term. Therefore, I am happy to let this Ph.D. who has the credentials and aptitude for this job do it for me, *do it for us*. Nigel is quite open to debating his choices with others, and, over the years, he has changed a number of these when other scholars have pointed out to him better choices which, nevertheless, met all of his criteria. In 1995, the Hunan Science & Technology Press brought out a revised, expanded version of this glossary under the title, *English-Chinese Chinese-English Dictionary of Chinese Medicine*. Although this is not actually a dictionary because it does not include definitions, it does include many changes and revisions in Wiseman's original terminology based on peer review and input.

The beauty of such a standard is that "one can have their cake and eat it too." If I don't like or agree with one of Wiseman's word choices, I can use my own, no problem. All I have to do is somehow note my divergence. This can be done with a footnote or some sort of commentary in brackets. In this case, all I have to say is that Wiseman's suggested term for this character is such and such. However, I prefer this or that for these or those reasons. Now the reader knows what the character in question is. How? By always being able to look it up in "Wiseman", but I can use my choice should I feel so brave to compete with this formidable linguist's knowledge.
At the moment, Wiseman's glossary is the only, freely available, professionally created, standard for translational terminology we have in the field of Chinese medicine besides Porkert's Latin. I believe it is very important for all English language translators to adopt this standard due to its many benefits, not least of which being that all our translations will use the same words for the same concepts. One of the great problems within our profession is that we never know if we are

talking about the same things since we all tend to use our own professional vocabularies. When you're talking about the glossy pulse and she is talking about the sliding pulse, A) is that the same as Dr. So-and-so's slippery pulse, and B) what is the original Chinese character?

Paradigm Publications should be publishing a true, clinical dictionary of Chinese medical terms by Nigel any time now. I say a true dictionary since it contains translations. When Western readers see the rationales for Nigel's word choices, I think there will be far less resistance to adopting his suggestions. They simply make too much sense.

Therefore, from here on out in this workbook, I will be using Nigel Wiseman's translational terminology, even though it sometimes sounds peculiar and infelicitous. When I disagree with one of Nigel's terms, I will footnote or otherwise note this divergence, and I strongly encourage other would-be Chinese medical translators to do the same.

12
Styles of Translation

In the mid-1950's, the great American sinologist, Edward H. Schafer, identified, two major styles of translating Chinese into English. He called these denotative and connotative.[1] In the thirteenth century in Tibet, scholars there also identified the same two broad styles of translation. In Tibetan, these are called *tsig gyur* and *don gyur*. *Tsig* means word and *gyur* means to translate. *Don* means meaning. Therefore, you can translate the words, word for word, or you can translate the meaning. Once you begin translating on your own, you will see that you cannot always do both at the same time. This is because languages are not identical in their logic, structure, grammar, and vocabulary. The closer two languages are to each other, the easier it is to translate the words *and* capture their intended meaning. The more dissimilar two languages are, the harder it is to capture both the words and their intended meaning in a single translation.

Now you might say, "So what, it's the meaning we're concerned with." And rightly so. But a translation of meaning is always a personal interpretation. It is So-and-so's opinion of the meaning. What if Dr. or Mr./Ms. So-and-so is wrong? Then maybe we do the wrong thing to the wrong person. If we are translating a poem or a novel and if our readers enjoy and are entertained by our translation, that may be all that is really necessary. But when it comes to the application of medical treatment, there is a whole other ethical dimension which must be taken into account. We need to have some way of checking the validity of a particular translator's interpretation.

In 1993, a group of American translators, editors, and publishers got together and formed the Council of Oriental Medical Publishers (COMP). One of the purposes for the founding of this trade organization was to create advertising labels which would identify for the reader the way in which a translation was done so that they could further judge its credibility and reliability in clinical practice. The members of COMP adopted Schafer's terms of denotative and connotative and added a third style or category of translation, functional translation.

Denotative translations

According to COMP's published guidelines, a translation may be labeled a denotative translation if it meets the following criteria.

1. The title of the source text, Chinese author, publisher, and edition must be stated. In other words, the translation is based on a known or identified foreign source text.

2. The translation must use a stated standard glossary for all Chinese medical technical terms. In other words, the choice of term translations should be made by formal philological means which are described somehow for the reader, such as in a translator's preface.

---

[1] Schafer, Edward H., "Non-translation and Functional Translation -- Two Sinological Maladies", *Far Eastern Quarterly*, Univ. of CA, 1954, p. 251-260

3. It needs to be a word for word translation which is as close to the original as possible so that, someone else using the stated glossary who was knowledgeable in Chinese would have a good chance of translating the text back into Chinese with a high degree of accuracy.

4. If the words themselves do not convey the meaning clearly and simply in understandable English, then the translator should either A) footnote this, B) add words which are not in the text in brackets or parentheses, or C) provide a commentary on the meaning.

These guidelines are pretty stringent. However, readers of a denotative translation can feel pretty confident that the work is an accurate if not elegant, verbatim translation which is as faithful as one language can be to a text originally in another language. Publisher members of COMP have agreed to label denotative translations as such on the bibliographic page of each appropriate book or published piece of material.

Connotative translations

Connotative translations are looser translations where the meaning of the words is emphasized over the words themselves. In a connotative translation, the translator is free to take more license in conveying what he or she thinks is the real or ultimate meaning of a text or passage. The translator still needs to identify the title of the Chinese text, author, publisher, and edition, but they do not need to use a stated, freely available standard glossary. Where the criteria of validity rests primarily with the source text in a denotative translation, the main criteria of validity in a connotative translation rests with the credentials of the translator. In other words, how do we know they are correct in their interpretation? Well, one way is their published credentials, where they studied Chinese, how long, their education in Chinese medicine, how long they have been in practice, etc.

Functional translations

Functional translations are COMP's loosest category of translation. The material presented is based on a Chinese language original or originals. However, the translator may choose to only present the parts or sections of the original which they think useful to their readership. In doing so, they do not necessarily need to inform their readers of exactly which sections of which pages of the Chinese original they have translated and which they have omitted. Further, this style of translation is even more connotative, perhaps rewording sentences or paragraphs entirely in order to simply convey certain technical information. Basically, this style of translation is more a gloss or a report *about* a Chinese original than a translation per se. As the "Draft Code for the Council of Oriental Medical Publishers" puts it, "These texts are freely abstracted paraphrases." As with connotative translations in general, the criteria of validity rests more with the translator's credentials than with the Chinese original, since there is no way to assess the translator's faithfulness to that original.

According to COMP guidelines, functional translations may use any technical terminology they choose. They do not need to be based on a stated, freely available standard glossary. However, translators of functional translations may choose to used such a stated standard glossary. In that case, the COMP designation would be functional translation using a standard translational terminology for Chinese medical technical terms. Blue Poppy Press's Recent Research Reports are examples of functional translations using Wiseman's terminology as their standard. They are more than mere abstracts, but they are not necessarily complete and unabridged translations of every sentence in the original Chinese articles.

Choosing a translational style

Which of the above three styles you choose to use when translating is up to you. A lot will depend on the purpose of your translation and whether it is for publication. If you are merely extracting information for use in your own clinical practice, you may only be jotting down the names of formulas and medicinals or acupuncture points.

However, when it comes to publication, I agree with Jürgen Kovacs in his "Linguistic Reflections on the Translation of Chinese Medical Texts" published in *Approaches to Traditional Chinese Medical Literature*. The Chinese medical literature is a type of *Fachprosa* or fact-prose. "*Fachprosa* are those texts that deal with science, technical issues, crafts, trade, administration, etc. and include such divergent categories as research reports, scientific textbooks, and administrative announcements, among others."[2] Because we are translating technical non-fiction whose implied instructions are meant to be put into real-life practice, I believe it is imperative that we maintain a high degree of faithfulness to the Chinese original. Therefore, I favor denotative translations of Chinese medical texts over connotative or functional translations. However, as stated above, we at Blue Poppy Press often do label our translations as functional. In this case, they are functional because we have chosen not to translate a source text in its entirety. Nevertheless, for the sections we have translated, we have used a standard translational terminology which is more denotative in its methodology than connotative.

---

[2] Kovacs, Jürgen, "Linguistic Reflections on the Translation of Chinese Medical Texts", *Approaches to Traditional Chinese Medical Literature*, ed. by Paul U. Unschuld, Kluwer Academic Publishers, Dordrecht, 1989, p. 86

13
Translating a Typical Section from a Modern Chinese Clinical Manual

As mentioned above, it is a good idea to start your translating by working on a section from a modern Chinese clinical manual. Such manuals typically are laid out in outline form. Much of the information conveyed is done so in lists and incomplete sentences which are virtually devoid of grammar. Such outlines and lists can be translated by simply using a Chinese-English dictionary. Since, as a clinician, this is probably the type of information you are looking for anyway, starting with this type of literature kills two birds with a single stone: A) you get the clinical information you need for your practice, while B) teaching yourself how to read modern medical Chinese.

The following section is taken from a modern Chinese book titled 现代难治病中医诊疗学 (*Xian Dai Nan Zhi Bing Zhong Yi Zhen Liao Xue, A Study of the Chinese Medical Diagnosis & Treatment of Modern Difficult to Treat Diseases*) by Wu Jun-yu and Bai Yong-bo, Chinese Medicine Ancient Books Publishing House, Beijing, 1993, pages 546-550. This section is on priapism. Basically, I know of nothing in the English language literature on Chinese medicine about this medical complaint. It may not be a commonly encountered complaint, but remember, our patients typically come to us for unusual complaints which other medicines have previously failed to fix. Therefore, compared to the typical Western medical general practitioner, we see a disproportionate number of patients with similarly unusual conditions.

First you will find the Chinese text reproduced in its entirety. After the text I then give a guide to its translation. Using this guide, one can orient oneself to other similar modern Chinese treatment manuals.

阴茎异常勃起

阴茎异常勃起是一种持续不消退的海绵体痛性勃起，其病理生理机制尚未完全清楚。近来认为是由于阴茎海绵体神经——动脉机制障碍所致，可由于血液性疾病、神经性疾病、机械性阻塞静脉回流、炎症以及药物使用不当等原因引起。治疗多采用镇静、冷敷、抗凝血、局部神经阻滞及手术分流等，效果不甚满意，有些可造成阳萎等继发性性功能障碍。

中医学称该症为"阳强"或"强中"。其病因为肾水亏乏，肝经火盛，或瘀血败精阻络，致宗筋损伤，阴纵不收。治疗多依据病因，或滋阴降火，或清肝泻热，或活血行瘀等，力使邪气得除，宗筋得润，纵挺之证得以缓解。

【西医诊断】

参考《实用男性学》[119]标准和《实用简明男性学》[120]定义。

1. 阴茎呈持续勃起状态，勃起可持续数小时、数日至数周，其勃起无性兴奋性和性欲要求，同时伴有疼痛与不适感。

2. 仔细询问病史及发病过程，注意有无外伤史、血液系统和神经系统疾病史、生殖系统感染史及有无使用血管扩张药物史等，初步判断其原因。

3. 做血细胞计数、血小板计数、血红蛋白电泳、尿三杯实验、尿液培养以及有关肿瘤的各项生化检验，进一步判明其原因，必要时可做阴茎海绵体血管造影，以明确诊断。

【中医诊疗】

阴茎异常勃起《内经》称为"纵挺不收"；隋·巢元方命名为"强中"；清·陈士择称为"阳强不倒"。认为其病因多为肾水内涸，虚火内炽，或肝经实火耗损阴精而致宗筋失养，纵挺不收。近来有不少医家认为除阴虚火旺以外，尚有瘀血、湿热、败精阻络等因素可引起该症，丰富了其治疗方法。

一　病因病机

阴茎异常勃起虽可由多种原因引起，但均与肝肾二经关系密切。肝脉绕阴器，主宗筋；肾主水，为藏精之所，开窍于二阴，肝肾失和即可致宗筋失养，阴茎纵挺不收则为其主要表现之一。临床上大致可分为以下几种情况：

1．阴虚火旺　素体阴虚，或恣情纵欲，房室过频，而致阴精内耗，相火妄动，阴不敛阳，则宗筋纵挺，坚硬不倒。

2．肝火内炽　情志不遂，肝气郁结，久而化火，内灼真阴。阴衰火盛，实邪循径下扰宗筋，可致阴茎坚挺不收。

3．败精阻窍　手淫过度，或房事频繁，忍精不泄，可致败精内滞，湿热内蕴，瘀阻窍道，经络失和，肝经气血运行不畅，宗筋失养，则阴茎不收。

4．药物劫阴　素体阳弱而过用强阳助火之剂，内耗阴精，则阳亢无制，宗筋纵挺不收。

5．血瘀络阻　阴器外伤，血溢络外，瘀血停聚，经脉闭阻，阴器周围血流不畅，败血瘀阻其间，致阴茎不收，坚硬如石。

二、四诊要点

（一）望诊

面红目赤为肝火炽盛；午后颧红为阴虚火旺；舌红苔黄多为肝热；舌红少苔多为虚火；舌质紫暗或有瘀斑为瘀血内阻；舌苔黄腻或白腻为败精湿热内阻；阴茎痛胀，皮色紫暗为瘀血阻络；阴囊潮热，或见白浊，为败精阻窍或肝胆火炽。

（二）闻诊

小溲短赤，气味臊臭为肝胆火炽，湿热下注；小溲短黄，不浑不臭为阴虚火旺。

（三）问诊

房事频繁，施泄无度者易致阴虚火旺；房事之时，忍精不泄者易致败精阻窍；外伤后发病者多为瘀血阻络；用药后发病者，多为药物伤阴；性欲素旺，病情屡发者为阴虚火旺或肝火内炽；小便黄赤短少为热盛或阴虚；小溲频数涩痛为败精湿热阻窍；阳强兼见胸胁胀满，烦急易怒为肝热；兼见腰痠膝软、潮热盗汗为阴虚。

（四）切诊

脉象弦数多为肝郁化火；细数多为肾阴亏虚；弦滑多为败精阻窍；沉涩多为血瘀阻络。

三、辨证论治

（一）证治要点

本病在临床上，原则上应针对导致宗筋弛缓、阳强不倒的阴虚火旺、肝胆火炽、药物劫阴，败精阻窍、瘀血阻络等不同病机，分别采用滋阴降火、清肝泻胆、活血化瘀、通精开窍，抑阳倒戈等方法，实者泻之，虚则补之，纠其偏颇，使邪去正扶，而宗筋弛缓、阳强不倒之症当可获愈。但还应掌握标本缓急，以灵活对待。一般说来，本病阴茎异常勃起，其实邪标症多属紧急，故在治疗时，应急则治标，以抑阳倒戈等为主要治法，其阴虚的一面，在急性期适当照顾即可，不应喧宾夺主，以免延误病情。而俟病情略有好转，治疗又应充分考虑其阴液耗伤之本，注意滋阴柔肝、缓急止痛，不可一味攻伐，以防进而劫阴耗液，致成变证。

（二）证治方法

1．阴虚火旺

辨证特征　阳强不倒，欲念难除，茎睾胀痛，头晕耳鸣，心烦少寐，腰膝痠软，舌质红少或薄黄、脉弦细数。

治疗方法　滋肾降火。

常用方知柏地黄丸。

2．肝火内炽

辨证特征　阴茎易举，持久不萎，面红目赤，两胁胀满，急躁易怒，溲黄便干。舌红苔黄，脉弦数。

治疗方法清肝泻火。

常用方　龙胆泻肝汤。

3．败精阻窍

辨证特征　阳强不倒，茎睾胀痛，小便赤涩疼痛频数，少腹拘急，阴囊潮湿、或见尿中白浊。舌质红，苔白中厚腻，脉弦滑。

治疗方法　通精开窍。

常用方　程氏萆薢分清饮。

4．药物劫阴

辨证特征　过用助阳药物后，阳强不倒，时久茎痛，勃起时并无性欲要求，睾丸坠胀，少腹拘急。舌质红，苔白，脉沉弦。

治疗方法　抑阳倒戈。

常用方　黄连猪肚丸。

5．瘀血阻络

辨证特征　外伤后阴茎举而不萎、肿胀疼痛、色紫暗，睾丸时痛，茎睾触之痛甚，舌质紫暗或有瘀斑，苔白，脉沉弦或沉涩。

治疗方法　活血定痛。

常用方　乳香定痛散。

四、专病专方

（一）中成药

1．知柏地黄丸　每次 1～2 丸，每日 2 次，温开水送下，对阴虚火旺型患者可有较为明显疗效。

2．龙肝泻肝丸　每次服 6 g，每日 2～3 次，温开水送下，对于肝火内炽型患者可有较好疗效。

（二）针灸

针行间、太冲、蠡沟、三阴交、阴陵泉，用泻法，毫针刺入，留针 3～5 分钟。

（三）气功

当欲火来潮时，身体放松，内视龟头部位，深吸气以意领气，至会阴，提谷道，入长强穴，气沿督脉直上至百会穴，下颏内收，呼气入脑，内视百会穴，反复呼吸运行。要求呼吸平静，做到缓、慢、细、长，一般呼吸 3～5 次即可平息欲火。身体姿势不限。

五、调护与预防

平素应积极参加健康文娱活动，保持身心愉快。建立正常性生活规律，适当节制房事，戒除手淫，避免不良性刺激。一旦患病，不要紧张，耐心治疗，并注意保持心情舒畅，避免郁怒伤肝。不宜过用壮阳之品。平素少食肥甘厚味，以免助湿生痰。

【诊疗参考】

一、中医辨证分型标准（参照《中医诊疗常规》[7]所载标准）

（一）诊断依据

1．同房射精后阴茎仍持续痛性勃起，历时数小时乃至数日不能自行疲软。

2．也可突然发生，未同房而阴茎自行挺勃，历久不衰。

3．常有平时耽嗜色欲，性欲亢进，频频行房史。

4．可有外伤腰髓，或为增进阳事自服燥热丹面药物史。

（二）辨证要点

1．肝经实热

（1）体质素壮，性欲亢进，同房后阴茎仍持续勃起，历时日而不衰萎，阴茎瘀血，色紫暗，胀痛。

（2）心烦不眠或常有恐惧感，或排尿困难，尿痛，口干口苦，大便秘结。

（3）舌苔黄，脉弦浮或数而有力。

2．阴虚火旺

（1）房室不节，色欲过度，或妄服升阳之药，阴茎勃起持久不衰，胀痛。

（2）形体消瘦，五心烦热或潮热，腰痠，头昏目眩，咽干口燥，大便秘结，小便黄赤涩痛，或有精液自溢。

（3）舌红少津，脉细数。

二、疗效判断标准（《中医诊疗常规》[7]所载标准）

1．痊愈：治疗后阴茎疲软，性功能正常。

2．无效：治疗后阴茎仍不能疲软。

三、名医诊疗特色

冷方南氏认为：阳强一病，有虚有实，实者有实火、湿热之分，虚乃阴虚阳亢而成。

其病位在肝。肝主筋，总宗筋之会，会于前阴，即阴茎之体也，肝之火邪下窜宗筋，而筋体被火热之灼炽痉挛，则阳强不倒，坚硬不衰，故用当归龙荟汤，大苦大寒之品，直泻肝火，濡润宗筋，更加白芍、甘草，名芍药甘草汤，专能缓解止痛，标本兼施，故病证可除矣。(冷方南主编. 中医男科临床治疗学. 第 1 版. 北京：人民卫生出版社，1991:66)

四、治疗参考

徐学军等报道：用蝮蛇抗栓酶 0.25u 加生理盐水 5ml 于阴茎海绵体内注射治疗阴茎异常勃起患者 5 例，注射后 20～30min 阴茎开始变软，勃起消退。随访 3～13 月未见复发，且性功能正常，全部治愈。〔男性学杂志1990；(4)：103〕

霰景春以芍药90ｇ，元参30ｇ，甘草60ｇ，水煎每日 1 剂治疗 1 例暴饮后同房致阳强不倒8天者，6剂即告痊愈，随访 1 年未复发，性生活正常。〔四川中医1988；(10)：21〕

张景祥以桃仁、红花、白芍各20ｇ，土鳖虫、荔枝核、木通、泽兰、甘草各10ｇ，没药8ｇ，大黄6ｇ，水煎服每日 1 剂，并加用血竭、大黄各10ｇ，锻自然铜6ｇ，冰片1ｇ，碾末加于面糊中，外涂于阴茎，治疗1例新婚阳强不倒3日者，2剂药后阴茎渐见松弛，8日后痊愈，未再复发。(冷方南主编. 中医男科临床治疗学. 第 1 版. 北京：人民卫生出版社，1991:70)

(陈文伯　陈　生)

The section heading in bold face (阴茎异常勃起) is the name of the disease. Below is a literal rendering of each word in this title.

阴 (*yin*, hidden, secret), 茎 (*jing*, stalk), 异 (*yi*, change, different), 常 (*chang*, normal), 勃 (*bo*, vigorous, thriving, exuberant), 起 (*qi*, stand up, arise), *i.e.*, yin stalk = penis, different from normal = abnormal, vigorous standing up = erection

At first, such a literal rendering may make no sense. However, we are supposed to be either students at a Chinese medical school or practicing professionals. This means we are supposed to have a good idea of Western medical terminology and disease categories. So we need to ask ourselves, is there any Western medical disease having to do with abnormal penile erections? Yes there is: priapism. This means abnormal, persistent erections without appropriate sexual stimulation. OK, is there any way we can be sure of this. Yes again. But to do so, we are going to need a Chinese-English *Western* medical dictionary. The name of one good one is found in the bibliography at the rear of this book. We have already looked up each character in the section title. So now we go to a Chinese-English medical dictionary and look up the Pinyin for this title in alphabetical order. In other words, we look up the first word *yin* (阴) and scan down till we find the second word *jing* (茎). Then we continue scanning down until we find the third word *yi* (异), the fifth word *chang* (常), the sixth word *bo* (勃), and finally the seventh word *qi* (起). Next to this should be the word priapism. Another, perhaps quicker way to check if your translational hunch is correct is to go to an English-Chinese Western medical dictionary. In that case, look up the English word priapism and see if the Chinese characters given in the English to Chinese dictionary tally. I can tell you, they will.

Next, under the bold-faced disease name, we see two paragraphs of fairly dense text. In most modern Chinese clinical manuals, these first introductory paragraphs have to do with the definition of the disease category. Paragraph number one is the Western medical definition of priapism. *You do not need to translate this*! You can get his information much quicker and more easily by going to *The Merck Manual.*

The second paragraph is the Chinese medical categorization of priapism. The first sentence says: "Chinese medicine calls this condition '阳强 (*yang qiang*, yang strong)' or '强中(*qiang zhong*, strong stroke).' In other words, priapism is a modern Western disease category. As such, it does not exist in the traditional Chinese medical literature. However, Chinese are just as likely to suffer from this condition as Westerners; so of course there is some equivalent of priapism in the traditional Chinese medical literature. Knowing that priapism was called *yang qiang* or *qiang zhong* allows us to go to a more traditional Chinese medical book and find this disease category in the table of contents. You might also want to look up the words *yang qiang* in Wiseman's *English-Chinese Chinese-English Dictionary of Chinese Medicine* in the Chinese to English section. There you will find *yang qiang bu dao* (阳强不倒 , persistent erection). Literally, this phrase says, "Yang strong (does) not reverse (invert, pour, move backward, etc.)"

Following the identification of priapism with *yang qiang*, the next sentence opens with the words, 其病因为. The first character means "its", the second means "disease", the third means "cause", and the fourth means "is": "Its disease causes are..." (Please look each of these up in your Chinese-English dictionary.) What follows then is a long sentence with a number of clauses set off by commas. Each of these clauses is a succinct enumeration of the disease causes of this condition. As a clinician, you definitely want to translate these. However, because these are going to be Chinese medical technical terms, you will need to look them up *twice*. First you need to look them up in your regular Chinese-English dictionary. Write down the Pinyin and write down the meaning of each individual word. Then look the Pinyin up in Wiseman's *English-Chinese Chinese-English Dictionary of Chinese Medicine*. Now you will have Wiseman's standard translation of these technical terms. The next sentence tells you the main treatment principles for treating this condition with Chinese medicine. Below I will give you my translation of this paragraph. But, please, translate it yourself first before reading mine. Practice, practice, practice.

Bob's translation:

Chinese medicine calls this condition '*yang qiang*' or '*yang zhong*.' Its disease causes are kidney water depletion and lack, liver channel fire exuberance, or static blood and vanquished essence obstructing the network vessels. This results in ancestral sinew (or the gathering of sinews, *i.e.,* the penis) detriment and damage. The yin (*i.e.,* penis) becomes erect (or upright) and is not restrained. Treatment (of this condition) is mostly based on the disease causes. (Therefore,) one might enrich water and downbear fire (in the case of kidney water debility and lack), clear the liver and drain heat (in the case of liver channel fire exuberance), or quicken the blood and move stasis (in the case of blood stasis obstructing the network vessels). By doing this, evil qi obtains dispelling and the ancestral sinews obtain moistening. Hence the condition of erection obtains relaxation and resolution.

In the above paragraph, words in parentheses have been added by me in order to bring out the meaning more fully. When done for publication, such added words are probably best done with brackets [ ], since some modern Chinese does include parentheses. You will also notice that I have broken up long sentences with many clauses into shorter English sentences. The norm for good, powerful English is to use short, active voice, declarative sentences in the following word order: subject, verb, object. Chinese sentences are often much longer and more complex. Personally, I do not feel the need of retaining that structural complexity and am willing to sacrifice that level of textual faithfulness to well written English.

If you looked up each word in the above paragraph separately, you took more time then you may have needed to and may have created some unnecessary conundrums for yourself. In Chinese, each character is its own word. But Chinese like to talk and, therefore, write in two word combinations. Such two word combinations form compound terms. In the above paragraph there are several such compound terms. For instance, 依 (*yi*) means "to depend on, to comply with, and according to". 据 (*ju*) means "to reside, dwell, be in, store up, lay by, and stay put". If you looked each of these words up separately, you may be perplexed on how to string them together in a meaningful way. However, if you look up the first word, *yi*, after its main definitions, there is a listing of two word compound terms beginning with this *yi*. These are in smaller type within bold-faced brackets. So, if you think that a character might be a compound term, you should scan down the listing of compound terms looking for the second character in the pair. When you find a match, A) you've saved yourself from looking up the second character, and B) you now know a compound term whose meaning may have been difficult to arrive at by simply adding the meanings of both individual words together.

Next we see the bold-faced heading 西医诊断 (*xi yi zhen duan*). *Xi* means "Western", *yi* means "medicine", and *zhen duan* is a compound term which means "diagnosis". Therefore, this heading says "Western medical diagnosis". *Do not translate this section.* First of all, it is likely to have Western medical jargon translated into Chinese. To translate this you will definitely need a Chinese-English *Western* medical dictionary. If you simply look each character up independently, you probably will wind up with gobbledy-gook. Secondly, why do this? Just look this kind of information up in *The Merck Manual.* Very commonly, that appears to be where Chinese authors get this kind of information in the first place. If you do translate it, it is often almost identical with that English language source.

The next bold faced section says 中医诊疗 (*zhong yi zhen liao*). *Zhong* means "center or central". The name for China in Chinese is *Zhong Guo*, the Central or Middle Country. *Yi* we know means "medicine". So *zhong yi* means "Chinese medicine". *Zhen* means "diagnosis" and *liao* means "treatment". Therefore, this heading says "Chinese medical diagnosis and treatment".

Under this heading, we see a rather text dense paragraph. In the first line of this paragraph, we see two characters in double chevrons: ⟪ 内经 ⟫. This says *Nei Jing* or *The Inner Classic.* These double chevrons are typically the way book titles are set off in modern Chinese texts. In any case, we know that this section is going to have something to do with the history of this disease in Chinese medicine. As a clinician, you may or may not be interested in this information. As a beginner, I'm going to suggest that you leave it alone. There are doctors' names and the names of dynasties which you might not recognize either A) as proper names or B) who or what they are.

Under this paragraph you will see the character for one (一). Next to it is the heading 病因病机. *Bing yin* we have already looked up and it means "disease causes". The third character is the same as the first. We already know it means "disease". The fourth character is *ji* and means "dynamic or mechanism". So this heading as a whole translates as "Disease causes, disease mechanisms." This is a very common heading in Chinese clinical manuals. You will see it all the time.

Under this heading, there is again a text dense paragraph. It has to do with the liver and kidney channels' relationship to the penis. It's interesting, but leave it for now. Then you will see Arabic numbers on the left-hand side, 1-5. Each number is followed by a relatively short sentence, not a long paragraph. As a practitioner or would-be practitioner, we need to know what are the disease causes and mechanisms of this disease, and this looks relatively short and sweet, in outline form. So let's go for it! Please look up the characters in the following five sections and see if you can string them together in a meaningful way. After you have done so, check your translation with mine.

Bob's translation:

1. Yin vacuity, fire effulgence: Habitual bodily yin vacuity or unbridled passion and indulgence of desire with excessively numerous bedroom affairs (*i.e.*, sex) may result in yin essence being consumed internally. (In that case,) ministerial fire may frenetically stir and yin fails to restrain yang. This leads to erection of the ancestral sinews (or gathering of sinews) which become hard and does not collapse.

2. Liver fire internally blazing: If (one's) emotions are not satisfied, liver qi may become depressed and bound. If this endures and transforms into fire, (this) may burn internally true yin. If yin becomes debilitated, fire becomes exuberant. Replete evils follow the channel (*i.e.*, the liver channel) to descend and harass the ancestral sinews. This can result in the yin stalk becoming hard and erect and are not restrained (gathered in, brought to an end, etc.).

3. Vanquished essence obstructing the orifices: Due to excessive hand looseness (*i.e.*, masturbation) or to numerous bedroom affairs in which the essence is born and not discharged (*i.e.*, repeated sexual intercourse without ejaculation), the essence may have become vanquished and internally stagnated. Damp heat internally brews and stasis obstructs the orifices and pathways. The channels and network vessels lose their harmony and the liver channel qi and blood's movement is not smooth (or easy). The ancestral sinews lose their nourishment and this results in the yin stalk not being restrained (brought to an end, gathered in, etc.).

4. Medicinal substances plunder yin: Habitual bodily yang weakness and overuse of yang-strengthening, fire-invigorating prescriptions internally consume yin essence leading to yang hyperactivity without control. The ancestral sinews become erect and are not restrained (brought to an end, gathered in, etc.)

5. Blood stasis network vessel obstruction: If the yin organs (*i.e.*, genitalia) are externally damaged, blood may spill over outside the network vessels. Static blood then collects (including the meaning of "stops") and gathers. The channels and vessels become blocked and obstructed and the blood flow peripheral to the yin organs is not smooth (or easy). Vanquished blood becomes static and obstructs the spaces between them resulting in the yin stalk not being restrained (brought to an end, gathered in, etc.) and hard like a rock.

Next we come to another Chinese number. Do you remember it? 二 means "two". This is followed by yet another number. 四 (*si*) means "four". 诊 (*zhen*) means "examination". *Si zhen*, therefore, means the "four examinations". 要 (*yao*) means "essential" and 点 (*dian*) means "point". So this next heading means, "the essential points of the four examinations." Then you will see the Chinese numbers 1-4, this time in parentheses. Each number is followed by two characters, the second of which is *zhen*, "examination". Therefore, it does not take rocket science to know that each of these four sections deals with the key points of one of the four examinations *vis à vis* this condition. This is OK stuff and is clinically relevant. But we are going to skip it nevertheless. Why? Because the next section says "Treatment Based on Pattern Discrimination", and under that section they *always* give the signs and symptoms of each pattern. So we actually do not need to translate this material. We are still going to get the signs and symptoms we need as clinicians. (Of course, if you do have the time and energy to translate this section, it certainly won't hurt you and it will help hammer home the key points and the logic of Chinese medicine.)

So now you should see 三 (*san*, three) followed by 辨证论治 (*bian zheng lun zhi*). *Bian* means "to discriminate". *Zheng* in this context means "pattern". *Lun* means "discussion, talk, treatise, view, opinion", etc., but here means "determine, based on, by, in terms of". *Zhi* means to "treat". In order to make the English of these four words sound correct to a native English-speaker, we have to change their word order: "Treatment based on pattern discrimination."

Next, we again have the number one in parentheses (一). This is followed by the words 证治要点 (*zheng zhi yao dian*, main points of pattern treatment). When we look at this section, we see a text dense paragraph. I say skip it, at least as a beginner. Everything you need to know as a clinician will be covered in the sections below. So we'll drop down to section number two (二) 证治方法 , *zheng zhi fang fa*. This means "pattern treatment methods". The last two characters separately mean "formula and method or technique" respectively. However, as a compound term, they can be simply rendered as "method".

Now we see Arabic numerals again — this time 1-5. Each of these is the name of a TCM pattern of this disease. Underneath the name of the pattern it says 辨证特征, *bian zheng te zheng*. *Bian zheng* we already know means "pattern discrimination". *Te zheng* is a compound term meaning "characteristics or trait". In most clinical manuals, this section is headed by the words 主证 (*zhu zheng*, ruling or main symptoms). There may or may not be a colon after this heading. In this case there is not. But what follows is a list of signs and symptoms. Although there is a period at the end of this list, it is not necessarily a complete sentence from the English point of view since it may not have a verb.

I will translate this section below so you can check your translation after you look up every word. But first I would simply like tell you what each subsection is since most modern Chinese clinical manuals follow this same general outline. So next we come to the words 治疗方法 (*zhi liao fang fa*). This means treatment method. In other books you might find simply 治法 (*zhi fa*, treatment methods) or 治则 (*zhi ze*, treatment principles). What follows is a listing of treatment principles for the pattern under discussion. Then it says 常用方 (*chang yong fang*, commonly used formula). Other books may only say 方 (*fang*) for formula, 方药 (*fang yao*) for formula and medicinals, or 处方 (*Chu fang*) for prescription. Here there is no colon, but many books will put in a colon followed by the name of the formula. This book does not give the ingredients of the formulas listed, but most will. In that case, either there will be a colon after the formula name followed by a listing of the ingredients or there will be another subheading, 组成 (*zu cheng*), composition. For each of the five patterns listed here there are the same three subheadings or categories of information: symptoms, treatment principles, and treatment. If it was an acupuncture or *tui na* book, this last section would either be acupuncture points or *tui na* manipulations at points or body parts.

Bob's translation:

1. Yin vacuity fire effulgence

Pattern discrimination characteristics: Persistent erection, desire and thoughts (of sex) hard to eliminate, penis and testes distended and painful, dizziness and tinnitus, heart vexation, scanty sleep, low back and knee aching and flaccidity, a red tongue body with scanty or thin, yellow fur, and a bowstring[1], fine, rapid pulse

Treatment methods: enrich the kidneys and downbear fire

Commonly used formula: *Zhi Bai Di Huang Wan* (Anemarrhena & Phellodendron Rehmannia Pills)

2. Liver fire internally blazing

Pattern discrimination characteristics: An easily erect penis which is erect for a long time and does not wilt, a red face and red eyes, bilateral rib-side distention and fullness, tension, agitation, and easy anger, yellow urination, dry stools, a red tongue with yellow fur, and a bowstring, rapid pulse

Treatment methods: Clear the liver and drain fire

---

[1] Wiseman's term for *xian mai* is a stringlike pulse. I prefer bowstring since the character has the bow radical in it and it does not mean a limp string, but only one drawn tight, like a bowstring or the string on a musical instrument.

Commonly used formula: *Long Dan Xie Gan Tang* (Gentiana Drain the Liver Decoction)

3. Vanquished essence obstructing the orifices

Pattern discrimination characteristics: Persistent erection, penis and testes distended and painful, urination red and astringent, aching and painful, frequent and numerous, lower abdominal cramping, scrotal tidal dampness (*i.e.*, sweating), the possible appearance of white turbidity within the urine, a red tongue body with white fur which is thick and slimy in the center, and a bowstring, slippery pulse

Treatment methods: Free the flow of the essence and open the orifices

Commonly used formula: Master Cheng's *Bie Xie Fen Qing Yin* (Dioscorea Hypoglauca Separate the Clear Drink)

4. Medicinal substances plunder yin

Pattern discrimination characteristics: After enduring use of yang-invigorating medicinals, there is persistent erection. Sometimes there is enduring penile pain. At the time of erection, there is no sexual desire or demand. The testes are sagging and distended and there is lower abdominal cramping. The tongue body is red with white fur, and the pulse is deep and bowstring.

Treatment methods: Repress yang and topple the dagger-axe[2]

Commonly used formula: *Huang Lian Zhu Du Wan* (Coptis Pig Tripe Pills)

5. Static blood obstructing the network vessels

Pattern discrimination characteristics: After external injury, the penis raises and does not wilt. There is swelling, distention, aching, and pain and its color is purple and dark. The testes may occasionally be painful and penile and testicular pain may be exceptionally severe. The tongue body is purple and dark or has static spots with white fur. The pulse is deep and bowstring or deep and choppy.

Treatment methods: Quicken the blood and stabilize the pain

Commonly used formula: *Ru Xiang Ding Tong San* (Frankincense Stabilize Pain Pills)

As you will see above, I sometimes had to make sentences where there were only phrases in Chinese. In other places, I ignored periods in the source text where they were not necessary. In particular, I'd like to draw your attention to two words which can be problematic for beginners. The first is 或 (*huo*). This can mean "perhaps, maybe, probably", or it may simply mean "or". In

---

[2] A dagger-axe is an ancient sort of weapon. Here the penis is being likened to a dagger similar in meaning to the vulgar English prick.

a list of signs and symptoms, it usually means either there is possibly this or that symptom or it means or. In the first case, it is used in English as an adjective; in the second case as a conjunction. Basically, you have to try out both possibilities and see which fits the context best. The second word is 时 (*shi*). It means time. It can be translated as "at the time of" or "sometime." Again, one must figure this out from context.

Next we come to section number four (四, 专病专方). *Zhuan* means "particular". Therefore, *zhuan bing* means "particular disease", while *zhuan fang* means "particular formulas", *i.e.*, specific formulas for this specific disease. Then we have the Chinese number one in parentheses (一). Next to that it says 中成药, *zhong cheng yao*. *Zhong* means "center", but in this case it is a contraction for *Zhong Guo*, China or Chinese. *Cheng* means "to accomplish, to succeed, to become, or turn into". However, it also means "ready-made". If *yao* means "medicine", then the compound term *cheng yao* means "ready-made medicine". Hence the three characters means "Chinese ready-made medicines" or what are commonly called Chinese patent medicines.

Then there is an Arabic numeral one and two. Please try to translate these short sections on your own. Then see how I translate these *after you have given it your best shot.*

Bob's translation:

1. *Zhi Bai Di Huang Wan* (Anemarrhena & Phellodendron Rehmannia Pills): (Take) 1-2 pills each time, two times each day, washed down with warm boiled water. (Literally, *kai shui* says open water, but it means boiled water.) For yin vacuity fire effulgence pattern, it can have a relatively marked therapeutic effect.

2. *Long Dan Xie Gan Wan* (Gentiana Drain the Liver Pills): Six grams each time, 2-3 times each day, washed down with warm boiled water. For liver fire internally blazing pattern, it can have a comparatively good therapeutic effect.

Next we come to the section on acupuncture. There is a Chinese character for the number two in parentheses (二). Next to it are the characters for acupuncture and moxibustion (针灸). Please try to translate the following acupuncture protocol and then check it against my rendition.

Bob's translation:

Needle *Xing Jian* (Liv 2), *Tai Chong* (Liv 3), *Li Gou* (Liv 5), *San Yin Jiao* (Sp 6), and *Yin Ling Quan* (Sp 9) using draining technique (or method). After puncturing and inserting a fine needle, retain the needles for 3-5 minutes.

(三), parentheses with the Chinese number three is followed by the words 气功 (*qi gong*). I've never tried to read anything in Chinese about *qi gong* and so I don't know any vocabulary associated with that art. That means that, should I wish to translate the following section, I would have to look up almost every word, and, then, I might not understand their contextual use. If you are interested in knowing the *qi gong* treatment of priapism, then be my guest.

Next you will see a Chinese number five (五) with a comma after it. The Chinese heading reads 调护. *Tiao hu* means "nursing or the care of a patient during convalescence". The next character (与) means "and" (*yu*). It is a conjunction. Then we have 预防 (*yu fang*), "prevention". So this section deals with the care during recuperation and prevention of this disease. It contains pretty *pro forma* advice about being careful to regulate and discipline one's sexual activity, not to masturbate, not to eat spicy, peppery, hot foods, not to get tense, and not to inappropriately or excessively use yang-invigorating ingredients. You can go ahead and translate it in its entirety if you want, but the contents of this passage are probably not going to be anything you don't already know or couldn't anticipate from the basic theories of Chinese medicine.

So, moving on, there are four bold-faced characters in brackets: 诊疗叁考 (*zhen liao can kao*). This means "special references for diagnosis and treatment". Looking at this section, notice the lines are short, the material is in outline form, and there is a lot of white space. This is good material for beginners. Give it a try. However, in terms of important clinically useful information, we have gotten the essence out of this chapter since we have learned the main patterns, their principles, and standard treatments (at least according to this book) of this condition.

At the very end of this section on priapism, you will note several characters in parentheses on the right-hand side. These are the names of the two authors of this section. They are 陈文伯, Chen Wen-bo, and 陈生, Chen Sheng.

Different clinical manuals may vary from the above outline in some particulars, but it is a very common pattern over all. As beginners, my advice is to scan a chapter in a clinical manual such as this, looking for the words 辨证论治 (*bian zheng lun zhi*, treatment based on pattern discrimination). Under that, you should see some numbers and text arranged in outline form. Next to each number, there will probably be four characters. In general, most Chinese authors like to use four characters when naming different patterns -- for instance: 肝郁气滞 (*gan yu qi zhi,* liver depression qi stagnation).

Under the pattern name, you should find a section on signs and symptoms, tongue and pulse. Then come the treatment principles or treatment methods. And then comes the treatment, be it a Chinese medicinal formula or a list of acupuncture points.

Some scholars may be aghast that I am suggesting to beginners not to translate sections of various works. This suggestion is not based on these sections being worthless or unimportant. Rather, it is based on my assessment of time-efficiency and cost-effectiveness. For beginners, the process of looking so many words up in a Chinese-English dictionary is very laborious and frustrating. One has to be careful at the beginning to focus on the most useful information which can be extracted most easily. As one's Chinese improves and one has to look up less and less characters, then one can tackle denser blocks of text which tend to have more and more complicated grammar. Here I am not saying that any material is worthless or unnecessary. I am only making a suggestion of how to prioritize one's translational endeavors as a beginner.

14
Translating a Typical Clinical Audit Report

Below is a sample of a typical Chinese clinical audit report appearing in Chinese TCM journals. If you understand some of the key words of this report, you will come across them again and again in other such articles. Please look up each Chinese character in this article in your Chinese-English dictionary. Please be sure to check to see if a character is followed by another character forming a compound term. If you think a character or characters is a technical Chinese medical term, then look these up in Wiseman's *English-Chinese Chinese-English Dictionary of Chinese Medicine*. After you have looked up each character in a sentence or section, then check my translation of that sentence or section to see how I have interpreted it.

(From *Yi Guan Jian Zhi Liao Jing Xing Tou Tong 148 Li, Hei Long Jiang Zhong Yi Yao*, #6, 1996, p. 38)

一贯煎治疗经行头痛 148 例

韩凤云

（天津市北辰医院）

笔者多年来，用一贯煎为主，加减治疗经行头痛 148 例，取得满意疗效，现报告如下：

1 临床资料

门诊病人 98 例，住院病人 50 例。年龄 15—25 岁，25 例；26—36 岁，38 例；39—49 岁，80 例；50 岁以上 5 例，病程 1—6 月，32 例；7—12 月，40 例；1—3 年，57 例；3—5 年，15 例；5 年以上，4 例。兼痛经者 28 例，兼发热者 12 例，兼呕吐者 37 例，兼情志异常者 13 例，兼经量过少者 34 例，兼经量过多者 24 例。

2 诊断标准

诊断标准，参照 1990 年内蒙古扎兰屯"全国中医第二次脑病会议"所制定的头痛诊断标准，并将此诊断标准应用范围扩大。

3 治疗方法

药物组成：沙参、麦冬、当归、生地、熟地各 20g，川楝子、鳖甲各 10g，枸杞子、阿胶各 20g，白芍 25g，鹿角霜、香附各 15g，加水适量，煎至，150ml，早晚分服；兼痛经进加益母草 30g，木香 12g；兼发热者加地骨皮 15g，丹皮 10g；兼呕吐者加半夏 10g，竹茹 15g，兼情志异常者加酸枣仁 15g，百合 25g；兼经量过多者加升麻 10g，黄芪 30g；兼经量过少者加太子参 20g，川芎 20g。

4 疗效评定标准

疗效评定标准参照 1986 年 6 月南通"第一次全国中医脑病工作会议"制定的疗效判定标准。

1、痊愈：临床症状消失，头痛及主要兼症消除，随访半年未复发。

2、好转：临床症状基本消失，头痛随访三个月未复发。

3、无效：临床症状治疗前后无改变。

5 治疗结果

治疗后不仅经行头痛得以痊愈或好转，其兼症均消失。痊愈 124 例，好转 22 例，无效 2 例。服药后 1—3 剂好转或痊愈者 85 例，4—6 剂好转或痊愈者 61 例，9 剂以上仍头痛 2 例，为无效。

6 典型病例

王某，女，42 岁，三年前恰值月经来潮，头痛加剧，口服"正痛片"、"脑宁"、"镇脑宁"等未效，口出秽语、打人毁物，被送至某院，行电击疗法，离院后遵医嘱长期口服奋乃静 4mgtid，安坦 4mgtid，二年未间断，一年前因故停药一周，又逢月经来临，症见：精神症状如初，头痛难忍，欲吐，经量减少，色淡，心悸，少寐，消瘦，舌淡、边有牡龈，脉细数无力。当拟滋阴养之法，方用一贯益加减。

处方：沙参、麦冬、当归、生地、熟地各20g，川楝子、鳖甲各10g，枸杞子、阿胶各20g，白芍25g，鹿角霜、香附各15g，百合25g，酸枣仁15g，浮小麦、生龙牡各30g。二剂，加水煎至200ml，分早中晚三次服用。二诊：神志清晰，头痛消失，月经量适中。

处方：原方减生龙齿、浮小麦、酸枣仁，二剂，煎服。三诊：月经结束，精神振作，面色红润，诸症消失。

又嘱，每于月经前一周口服人参归脾丸，早晚各一付、至月经来潮，连服三月。二年后随访，至今未发作。

7　体会

"脑为髓之海"。有赖肝脾肾之精血濡养之，以输布气血津液于头部，该患者禀赋虚弱，加之后天化源不足；适值经期前后阴血下注胞宫，精血益虚，髓海不足，脑髓失养而痛。又因阴血内亏，心神失养，神无所主，故有神志异常。上述诸药使用，共奏滋阴养血，补虚止痛之法。

The title of this article is: "*Yi Guan Jian* (One Linking Decoction) in the Treatment of 148 Cases of Menstrual Movement Headache." Notice that I have had to rearrange the word order in order to make my translation sound more "normal" in English. Literally, the Chinese text says: "*Yi Guan Jian* treatment menstrual movement headache 148 cases."

Under the title comes the author's name: Han Feng-yun. Literally, this means Han Wind-cloud. My guess is that this is a man's name, but this is not always easy for a non-Chinese to determine. Under the name there are some characters in parentheses. These are the author's work unit: the Tianjing Municipal Bei Chen Hospital. The character 市 (*shi*) means "market". But when it appears with a city name, it means "municipal or municipality". 北 (*bei*) means "north", and 辰 (*chen*) means "a celestial body". It is also the name of a traditional Chinese two hour "hour." In addition, it can also mean "time, day, or occasion". Here, I am not exactly sure how to translate this name. It may mean North Star. I am also ok with leaving it in Chinese as a proper name, similar to Shanghai or Beijing. 医院 (*yi yuan*) means hospital.

The text begins with a preamble or introduction. It says: "For many years, the author has mainly used *Yi Guan Jian* with additions and subtractions in the treatment of 148 cases of menstrual movement headache. This (protocol) has gotten satisfactory therapeutic effects, the report (of which) is as below:" This is a pretty standard introduction. Please make note of the characters for author (笔, *bi*), which literally means the noun "pen" or the verb "to write". Here it means "the writer". Also make note of the compound terms 满意 (*man yi*, satisfactory), 治效 (*zhi xiao*, therapeutic effects), 报告 (*bao gao,* to make a report), and 如下 (*ru xia*, as below or as follows).

Next you will see the bold-faced Arabic numeral 1 followed by the words, 临床资料 (*lin chuang*, clinical, *zi liao*, data). Therefore, literally, this heading means "clinical data". Actually, what follows is what we would call the cohort description in a Western scientific report. You will have to decide how you want to translate this. If you are doing a denotative translation, then you will have to say "clinical data". If you are doing a connotative or functional translation, then it is OK to say "cohort description", since that is what follows.

Following this heading, you have a series of essentially incomplete sentences separated by periods. 门诊 (*men zhen*) literally means "door examination". 病人 (*bing ren*) means "sick person". However, as a compound term, these four characters together mean simply "out-patient". Then you see the Arabic numerals 98 followed by the character 例 (*li*) which means "cases". So this first phrase says: "There were 98 out-patients." 住 (*zhu*) means "to reside or stay". Therefore, 住院病人(*zhu yuan bing ren*) means "in-patient". Thus, "There were 50 in-patients." 年龄 (*nian ling*) means "age". So, "There were 25 cases who were 15-25 years of age, 38 cases who were 26-36 years old, 80 cases who were 39-49 years of age; and five cases who were over 50 years of age." 病程 (*bing cheng*) means "disease duration". Therefore, the following lines read: "There were 32 cases whose disease duration or course was 1-6 months, 40 cases of 7-12 months, 57 cases of 1-3 years, 15 cases of 3-5 years, and four cases (whose disease had lasted) for over five years." The character 兼 (*jian*) means "simultaneously". So, "There were 28 cases with simultaneous painful menstruation, 12 cases with simultaneous fever, 37 cases with simultaneous vomiting, 13 cases with simultaneous emotional abnormality, 34 cases with simultaneous excessively scanty menstruation, and 24 cases with excessively profuse menstruation." Can you follow the logic of how I made these interpretations?

Now you come to the bold-faced Arabic numeral 2. The characters read 诊断标准 (*zhen duan*, diagnosis, *biao zhun*, criteria). Therefore, this heading means, "The diagnostic criteria." In other words, what follows is a recounting of the criteria used for the diagnostic inclusion of patients in this report. The paragraph reads, "The diagnostic criteria referred to were those diagnostic criteria established for headache by the 1990 Inner Mongolia (*i.e.*, a province in China) Zha Lan Tun (this appears to be a place name in Inner Mongolia) 'All National Chinese Medicine Second Brain Disease Conference' combined with other diagnostic criteria used in order to expand their scope." This is a complex sentence! Were you able to follow how I interpreted the words? You have got to rearrange the word order in order to make it sound normal in English. Frankly, as a Western clinician, this paragraph is not all that meaningful and may not have been worth the time puzzling it out. On the other hand, it is good to know that there were definite, written diagnostic criteria of inclusion in this study. Usually such diagnostic criteria have to do with the Western disease diagnosis, but sometimes they may explain how the pattern discrimination was made.

The heading beginning with a bold-faced Arabic numeral 3 says, 治疗方法 (*zhi liao fang fa*). 治疗(*zhi liao*) means "treatment" and 方法 (*fang fa*) means "method". Therefore, this heading says, "Treatment methods." Now we are to the meat of this discussion in terms of what clinicians are looking for, *i.e.*, effective treatment protocols. By the way, if we are doing a connotative or functional translation, we might have chosen to translate this section as "treatment protocol".

药物 (*yao wu*) means medicinal "substances". 咨成 (*zu cheng*) means "composition". What follows the colon is "the medicinal composition or prescription". In order to translate the majority of medicinal names in the following list, look up only the first character. Then turn to chapter 15 and find the Pinyin list of medicinal identifications. Find the first syllable in the alphabetized Pinyin list and then scan the character list alongside to match up the second character. This way you only have to look up the first character and then cut to this cheat sheet to find the second character.

Bob's translation:

Medicinal composition: Radix Glehniae Littoralis (*Sha Shen*), Tuber Ophiopogonis Japonici (*Mai Dong*), Radix Angelicae Sinensis (*Dang Gui*), uncooked Radix Rehmanniae (*Sheng Di*), cooked Rehmanniae (*Shu Di*), 20g @, Fructus Meliae Toosendan (*Chuan Lian Zi*), Carapax Amydae Sinensis (*Bie Jia*), 10g @, Fructus Lycii Chinensis (*Gou Qi Zi*), Gelatinum Corii Asini (*E Jiao*), 20g @, Radix Albus Paeoniae Lactiflorae (*Bai Shao*), 25g, Cornu Degelatinum Cervi (*Lu Jiao Shuang*), Rhizoma Cyperi Rotundi (*Xiang Fu*), 15g @. Add a suitable amount of water and boil down to 150ml. Administer in divided (doses) morning and evening. If there was simultaneous painful menstruation, Herba Leonuri Heterophylli (*Yi Mu Cao*), 30g, and Radix Auklandiae Lappae (*Mu Xiang*), 12g, were added. If there was simultaneous fever, Cortex Radicis Lycii Chinensis (*Di Gu Pi*), 15g, and Cortex Radicis Moutan (*Dan Pi*), 10g, were added. If there was simultaneous vomiting, Rhizoma Pinelliae Ternatae (*Ban Xia*), 10g, and Caulis Bambusae In Taeniis (*Zhu Ru*), 15g, were added. If there were simultaneous emotional abnormalities, Semen Zizyphi Spinosae (*Suan Zao Ren*), 15g, and Bulbus Lilii (*Bai He*), 25g, were added. If there was simultaneous profuse menstruation, Rhizoma Cimicifugae (*Sheng Ma*), 10g, and Radix Astragali Membranacei (*Huang Qi*), 30g, were added. And if there was simultaneous scanty menstruation, Radix Pseudostellariae (*Tai Zi Shen*), 20g, and Radix Ligustici Wallichii (*Chuan Xiong*), 20g, were added.

Note the use of the past tense in the above several sentences. This is a report of what the author did at some time in the past. Therefore, it needs to be written in past tense, although there is no tense in the Chinese *per se*.

Bold-faced heading Arabic numeral number 4 reads：疗效评定标准 (*liao xiao ping ding biao zhun*). This means, "Criteria for the assessment of the therapeutic effect." Under this heading we find the statement, "The assessment (or definition) of therapeutic effect were based on those established at the June, 1986 "First All National Chinese Medicine Brain Disease Working Meeting." Note I have chosen to leave out the repetition of the phrase, "definition of therapeutic criteria," in order to make a more normal-sounding English sentence.

Below this we again see non-bold-faced Arabic numerals 1-3. Each of these numerals is followed by a two character phrase. These read respectively: 1. cure, 2. turn for the better or improvement, and 3. no effect. After the words meaning "cure", we see that, "The clinical symptoms disappeared, the headache and the main simultaneous (or accompanying) symptoms were eliminated, and there was no recurrence on follow-up after half a year." After the words meaning "turn for the better", we read, "The clinical symptoms basically disappeared and there was no recurrence of headache on follow-up after three months. And after the words meaning "no effect", we find, "There was no change in the clinical symptoms from before to after treatment." The words in this last sentence require the most jiggling in order to make them sound like a native English-speaker's. Literally, the sentence reads, "Clinical symptoms treatment before/after no change."

Now we go on to the heading: 治疗结果 (*zhi liao jie guo*, treatment results or outcomes). This following paragraph tells us the outcomes or the results of the treatment. The paragraph says:

After treatment, not only the menstrual movement headache obtained cure or improvement but also the simultaneous (or accompanying) symptoms all disappeared. Cured: 124 cases, improved, 22 cases, and no effect, 2 cases. After administered 1-3 *ji*, 85 cases either improved or were cured. After 4-6 *ji*, 61 cases improved or were cured. After nine *ji* or more, two cases still had headache and there was no effect.

The word 剂(*ji*) is a measure word for pharmaceutical or other chemical preparations. When Chinese count objects, they just don't say one, two, three, etc. Rather, they add certain measure words depending on what is being counted. When learning to speak Chinese, it can be difficult to remember the right measure word when saying that you want two or these or three of those. Some translators translate this term as dose. However, this is not correct, since one *ji* usually refers to one packet of medicinals which are given in 2-3 divided doses per day. Therefore, I choose to leave this word in Pinyin and footnote its meaning the first time it is used, explaining the difficulties of translating it. It is one of the few words which English-speaking practitioners of Chinese medicine should probably just memorize, the same way we do not try to translate the word "qi".

Section six, headed by a bold-faced Arabic number 6, says: 典型病例 (*dian xing bing li*). This means a typical disease case. We might want to connotatively or functionally gloss that as a typical case history. In the paragraph below this heading, the first two words are the patients name. The first character is the surname Wang. The second character is 某 (*mou*). It means "certain or some". Therefore, rather than being the patient's complete name, this construction means "a certain Wang" or "some Wang." This is in order to preserve patient confidentiality. In other case histories, we might see Wang followed by two letter x's (王 x x), or, in other words, Wang Something-something. The next character is the word for woman. It means that the patient was female. Then comes the Arabic number 42 followed by the word for age. So the patient was 42 years old. Then we go into the present case history.

Bob's translation:

For three years, just before her menses came like a tide, her headache was aggravated. She had taken orally "*Zheng Tong Pian* (Correcting Pain Tablets)", "*Nao Ning* (Brain Quieter)", "*Zhen Nao Ning* (Settle the Brain Quieter)", and other (such ready-made medicines) without effect. From her mouth would exit foul speech. She would hit people and destroy things. She was arrested and taken to a certain hospital where she received electro-shock therapy. After leaving that hospital, she obeyed the doctor's advice to orally take perphenazine, 4mg three times per day, and artane, 4mg three times per day, for a long time. For two years she had not discontinued this. In the previous one year, due to a reason (*i.e.*, intentionally or willfully) had stopped the medicines completely. Again it followed that, just as her menses were about to come, the (following) symptoms were seen: her essence spirit (*i.e.*, mental-emotion) symptoms were like initially, the headache was difficult to bear, and she desired to vomit. The volume of her menstruate was reduced and scanty and it was pale in color. There were heart palpitations, reduced sleep, emaciation, a pale tongue with marks of the teeth on its sides, and fine, rapid, forceless pulse. Therefore, the treatment methods were to enrich yin with the nourishing method. The formula used was *Yi Guan Jian* with additions and subtractions.

In the previous paragraph, there are a number of difficult translational problems. First off, the woman had taken some presumably over-the-counter medications. The problem is whether to just give their Pinyin romanization or translate their names. I have chosen to do both. Then, for the phrase, 电击疗法 (*dian ji liao fa*), my Chinese-English medical dictionary gives sideration, fulguration, electric desiccation. The term *dian ji* means lightning stoke. This means that literally, we are talking about lightning stroke therapy. The patient was quite emotionally disturbed. So thinking what kind of therapy she might have been given, it seems probable that she received electro-shock therapy. Further down, the names of two Western medicines are given. The first one I found in Chinese-English dictionary, but I had to find the second one in my Chinese-English medical dictionary.

The next block of text begins with the words 处方 (*chu fang*) which mean "to write a formula" or, as a noun, "a prescription". Here's my translation of this prescription:

Prescription: Radix Glehniae Littoralis (*Sha Shen*), Tuber Ophiopogonis Japonici (*Mai Dong*), Radix Angelicae Sinensis (*Dang Gui*), uncooked Radix Rehmanniae (*Sheng Di*), and cooked Radix Rehmanniae (*Shu Di*), 20g @, Fructus Meliae Toosendan (*Chuan Lian Zi*) and Carapax Amydae Sinensis (*Bie Jia*), 10g @, Fructus Lycii Chinensis (*Gou Qi Zi*) and Gelatinum Corii Asini (*E Jiao*), 20g @, Radix Albus Paeoniae Lactiflorae (*Bai Shao*), 25g, Cornu Degelatinum Cervi (*Lu Jiao Shuang*) and Rhizoma Cyperi Rotundi (*Xiang Fu*), 15g @, Bulbus Lilii (*Bai He*), 25g, Semen Zizyphi Spinosae (*Suan Zao Ren*), 15g, Fructus Levis Tritici Aestivi (*Fu Xiao Mai*) and uncooked Dens Draconis & Concha Ostreae (*Long Mu*), 30g @. Two *ji* (were prescribed) to be added to water and decocted until 200ml (remained). This was then to be taken in divided doses, three times, morning, noon, and night. Second examination (*i.e.*, second visit): (The patient's) mind was clear, her headache had disappeared, and her menstrual volume was suitably medium or moderate.

Prescription: Uncooked Dens Draconis (*Long Chi*), Fructus Levis Tritici Aestivi (*Fu Xiao Mai*), and Semen Zizyphi Spinosae (*Suan Zao Ren*) were subtracted from the original formula and two (more) *ji* were boiled and administered. Third examination: Her menses had concluded, her essence spirit was bestirred (*i.e.*, vigorous), her facial color (or complexion) was red and moist, and all her symptoms had disappeared.

Again she was advised that one week before each menstruation she take orally *Ren Shen Gui Pi Wan* (Ginseng Restore the Spleen Pills), one hand(ful) morning and evening, until her menses had come like a tide and (that she should) continue taking this for three months. On follow-up two years later, up to the present there had been no recurrence.

Next you will see the bold-faced Arabic numeral 7. Next to it are the words 体会 (*ti hui*). This means "knowledge based on experience". One might gloss the meaning of this heading as "discussion or commentary", but this would loose the actual Chinese emphasis on the fact that the following is not just idle rationalization but is founded on the author's real-life experience.

Bob's translation:

"The brain is the sea of marrow." It is dependent on the moistening and nourishing of the essence and blood or the liver, spleen, and kidneys which transport the qi, blood, fluids, and humors to the head region. This patient's natural endowment was vacuous and weak. In addition, her latter heaven source of transformation was insufficient. It is appropriate that before and after the menstrual period, yin and blood descend and pour down to the uterus. If the essence and blood (thus) become all the more vacuous and the sea of marrow becomes insufficient. The brain marrow loses its nourishment and there is pain. It may also be due to yin blood internally depleted. The heart spirit (thus) loses its nourishment and the spirit has no place from which to be engendered. Therefore the mind becomes abnormal. The above stated medicinals when used together achieve the methods of enriching yin and nourishing the blood, supplementing vacuity and stopping pain.

As stated above, this article is fairly representative of the outline and common vocabulary of modern Chinese clinical audits. Therefore, you should memorize the meanings of the compound terms in the bold-faced headings. You should also try to memorize such common vocabulary as 处方 (*chu fang*), 治疗 (*zhi liao*), 药物 (*yao wu*, medicinal substances), 组成 (*zu cheng*, composition), 例 (*li*, case), 剂 (*ji*, measure word for medicinals), etc. In Appendix 2, there are several more journal articles like this to try to translate.

15
Short Cuts & Tricks of the Trade

There are a number of short cuts and tricks of the trade when it comes to translating modern medical Chinese. As a beginner, even under the best of circumstances, this is a laborious, time-consuming project. Therefore, any way to save some time is usually a good idea. One way to do that is to use what I call "cheat sheets." Cheat sheets are alphabetized lists of compound terms. You look up the first character to find out its Pinyin romanization. Then you scan down your alphabetized cheat sheet until you match up the second character. This way, you only have to look up the first character in your Chinese-English dictionary.

When I first developed this idea of cheat sheets, Nigel Wiseman had yet to publish his *English-Chinese Chinese-English Dictionary of Chinese Medicine*. In the Chinese to English section of that glossary, you will find both Chinese medicinals and acupuncture point names, all alphabetized by Pinyin. So, in reality, all you need is this glossary of Nigel's for "one stop shopping." However, these Chinese medicinals and acupuncture point names are mixed in with everything else. Therefore, I still like to use my cheat sheets for Chinese medicinals and acupuncture names. I find them a little bit faster than flipping through Nigel's whole book.

Acupuncture points

All publisher members of COMP have agreed to use *A Proposed Standard International Acupuncture Nomenclature: Report of a WHO Scientific Group*, World Health Organization, Geneva, 1991, as our standard for identifying acupuncture points. That being said, we all also agreed that, having stated our standard, we each would probably diverge from that standard in some way. The following are the channel name abbreviations suggested by the WHO:

Lung = LU

Large intestine = LI

Stomach = ST

Spleen = SP

Heart = HT

Small intestine = SI

Bladder = BL

Kidney = KI

Pericardium = PC

Triple burner = TE

Gallbladder = GB

Liver = LV

Governing vessel = GV

Conception vessel = CV

The rationale for this approach is that each abbreviation is two letters and each letter is capitalized. At Blue Poppy, we choose to diverge from this standard by changing:

LU to Lu

ST to St

SP to Sp

HT to Ht

KI to Ki

PC to Per

TE to TB

LV to Liv

Typically, we explain these divergences in the Preface to any of our books containing point names. Our convention at BPP Inc. is to give the Pinyin name first in italics followed by the channel abbreviation and standard number in parentheses — for instance: *Tai Chong* (Liv 3), *Xing Jian* (Liv 2), *Zu San Li* (St 36), *Nei Guan* (Per 6), etc. Nigel Wiseman does give actual English language translations of all acupuncture point names in his glossary besides this standard point numbering convention.

For all extra-channel extraordinary points (外经奇穴, *wai jing qi xue*), we recommend using O'Connor & Bensky's *Acupuncture: A Comprehensive Text* since this book is readily available in the U.S. and has the most complete listing of extra points with a standard practical notation system.

Readers should note that many acupuncture points have more than a single name. The names listed below are, in my experience as a translator, the most commonly occurring ones. For a fuller listing of acupuncture names and numbers, see Wiseman's *English-Chinese Chinese-English Dictionary of Chinese Medicine*.

八风	*Ba Feng*	(M-LE-8)		大敦	*Da Dun*	(Liv 1)
八邪	*Ba Xie*	(M-UE-2)		大赫	*Da He*	(Ki 12)
白环酚	*Bai Huan Shu*	(Bl 30)		大横	*Da Heng*	(Sp 15)
百会	*Bai Hui*	(GV 20)		大巨	*Da Ju*	(St 27)
胞肓	*Bao Huang*	(Bl 53)		大陵	*Da Ling*	(Per 7)
本神	*Ben Shen*	(GB 13)		大杼	*Da Zhu*	(Bl 11)
髀关	*Bi Guan*	(St 31)		大迎	*Da Ying*	(St 5)
臂臑	*Bi Nao*	(LI 14)		大钟	*Da Zhong*	(Ki 4)
秉风	*Bing Feng*	(SI 12)		大椎	*Da Zhui*	(GV 14)
步廊	*Bu Lang*	(Ki 22)		带脉	*Dai Mai*	(GB 26)
不容	*Bu Rong*	(St 19)		胆囊	*Dan Nang*	(M-LE-23)
长强	*Chang Qiang*	(GV 1)		胆俞	*Dan Shu*	(Bl 19)
承扶	*Cheng Fu*	(Bl 36)		地仓	*Di Cang*	(St 4)
承光	*Cheng Guang*	(Bl 6)		地机	*Di Ji*	(Sp 8)
承浆	*Cheng Jiang*	(CV 24)		地铄	*Di Wu Hui*	(GB 42)
承筋	*Cheng Jin*	(Bl 56)		定喘	*Ding Chuan*	(M-BW-1)
承灵	*Cheng Ling*	(GB 18)		犊鼻	*Du Bi*	(St 35)
承满	*Cheng Man*	(St 20)		督俞	*Du Shu*	(Bl 16)
承泣	*Cheng Qi*	(St 1)		兑端	*Dui Duan*	(GV 27)
承山	*Cheng Shan*	(Bl 57)		耳和	*Er He Liao*	(TB 22)
尺泽	*Chi Ze*	(Lu 5)		二间	*Er Jian*	(LI 2)
冲门	*Chong Men*	(Sp 12)		耳门	*Er Men*	(TB 21)
冲阳	*Chong Yang*	(St 42)		肺俞	*Fei Shu*	(Bl 13)
次髎	*Ci Liao*	(Bl 32)		飞杨	*Fei Yang*	(Bl 58)
大包	*Da Bao*	(Sp 21)		风池	*Feng Chi*	(GB 20)
大肠俞	*Da Chang Shu*	(Bl 25)		风府	*Feng Fu*	(GV 16)
大都	*Da Du*	(Sp 2)		丰隆	*Feng Long*	(St 40)

风门	*Feng Men*	(Bl 12)		脊中	*Ji Zhong*	(GV 6)
风市	*Feng Shi*	(GB 31)		颊车	*Jia Che*	(St 6)
腹哀	*Fu Ai*	(Sp 16)		肩井	*Jian Jing*	(GB 21)
浮白	*Fu Bai*	(GB 10)		建里	*Jian Li*	(CV 11)
附分	*Fu Fen*	(Bl 41)		肩髎	*Jian Liao*	(TB 14)
腹结	*Fu Jie*	(Sp 14)		肩内陵	*Jian Nei Ling*	(M-UE-48)
复溜	*Fu Liu*	(Ki 7)		肩前	*Jian Qian*	(M-UE-48)
府舍	*Fu She*	(Sp 13)		间使	*Jian Shi*	(Per 5)
扶突	*Fu Tu*	(LI 18)		肩外俞	*Jian Wai Shu*	(SI 14)
伏兔	*Fu Tu*	(St 32)		肩髃	*Jian Yu*	(LI 15)
浮邪	*Fu Xi*	(Bl 38)		肩贞	*Jian Zhen*	(SI 9)
跗阳	*Fu Yang*	(Bl 59)		肩中俞	*Jian Zhong Shu*	(SI 15)
肝俞	*Gan Shu*	(Bl 18)		角孙	*Jiao Sun*	(TB 20)
膏肓俞	*Gao Huang Shu*	(Bl 43)		交信	*Jiao Xin*	(Ki 8)
隔关	*Ge Guan*	(Bl 46)		解溪	*Jie Xi*	(St 41)
隔俞	*Ge Shu*	(Bl 17)		金津	*Jin Jin*	(M-HN-20)
公孙	*Gong Sun*	(Sp 4)		金门	*Jin Men*	(Bl 63)
关冲	*Guan Chong*	(TB 1)		筋缩	*Jin Suo*	(GV 8)
关门	*Guan Men*	(St 22)		京骨	*Jing Gu*	(Bl 64)
关元	*Guan Yuan*	(CV 4)		睛明	*Jing Ming*	(Bl 1)
关元俞	*Guan Yuan Shu*	(Bl 26)		经渠	*Jing Qu*	(Lu 8)
光明	*Guang Ming*	(GB 37)		鸠尾	*Jiu Wei*	(CV 15)
归来	*Gui Lai*	(St 29)		巨骨	*Ju Gu*	(LI 16)
颔厌	*Han Yan*	(GB 4)		巨阙	*Ju Que*	(CV 14)
合谷	*He Gu*	(LI 4)		居髎	*Ju Liao*	(GB 29)
禾髎	*He Liao*	(LI 19)		巨髎	*Ju Liao*	(St 3)
合阳	*He Yang*	(Bl 55)		绝骨	*Jue Gu*	(GB 39)
横骨	*Heng Gu*	(Ki 11)		厥阴俞	*Jue Yin Shu*	(Bl 14)
后顶	*Hou Ding*	(GV 19)		孔最	*Kong Zui*	(Lu 6)
后溪	*Hou Xi*	(SI 3)		库房	*Ku Fang*	(St 14)
华盖	*Hua Gai*	(CV 20)		昆仑	*Kun Lun*	(Bl 60)
滑肉门	*Hua Rou Men*	(St 24)		阑尾	*Lan Wei*	(M-LE-13)
华陀夹脊	*Hua Tuo Jia Ji*	(M-BW-35)		劳宫	*Lao Gong*	(Per 8)
环跳	*Huan Tiao*	(GB 30)		历兑	*Li Dui*	(St 45)
肓门	*Huang Men*	(Bl 51)		蠡沟	*Li Gou*	(Liv 5)
肓俞	*Huang Shu*	(Ki 16)		梁门	*Liang Men*	(St 21)
会阳	*Hui Yang*	(Bl 35)		梁丘	*Liang Qiu*	(St 34)
会阴	*Hui Yin*	(CV 1)		廉泉	*Lian Quan*	(CV 23)
会宗	*Hui Zong*	(TB 7)		列缺	*Lie Que*	(Lu 7)
魂门	*Hun Men*	(Bl 47)		灵道	*Ling Dao*	(Ht 4)
急脉	*Ji Mai*	(Liv 12)		灵台	*Ling Tai*	(GV 10)
箕门	*Ji Men*	(Sp 11)		灵墟	*Ling Xu*	(Ki 24)
极泉	*Ji Quan*	(Ht 1)		漏谷	*Lou Gu*	(Sp 7)

颅息	*Lu Xi*	(TB 19)	日月	*Ri Yue*	(GB 24)
络却	*Luo Que*	(Bl 8)	乳根	*Ru Gen*	(St 18)
眉冲	*Mei Chong*	(Bl 3)	乳中	*Ru Zhong*	(St 17)
命门	*Ming Men*	(GV 4)	三间	*San Jian*	(LI 3)
目窗	*Mu Chang*	(GB 16)	三蕉俞	*San Jiao Shu*	(Bl 22)
脑户	*Nao Hu*	(GV 17)	三阳络	*San Yang Luo*	(TB 8)
脑会	*Nao Hui*	(TB 13)	三阴	*San Yin Jiao*	(Sp 6)
脑空	*Nao Kong*	(GB 19)	上关	*Shang Guan*	(GB 3)
臑俞	*Nao Shu*	(SI 10)	上巨虚	*Shang Ju Xu*	(St 37)
内关	*Nei Guan*	(Per 6)	上廉	*Shang Lian*	(LI 9)
内庭	*Nei Ting*	(St 44)	上髎	*Shang Liao*	(Bl 31)
膀胱俞	*Pang Guang Shu*	(Bl 28)	商丘	*Shang Qiu*	(Sp 5)
脾俞	*Pi Shu*	(Bl 20)	商曲	*Shang Qu*	(Ki 17)
偏历	*Pian Li*	(LI 6)	上腕	*Shang Wan*	(CV 13)
魄户	*Po Hu*	(Bl 42)	上星	*Shang Xing*	(GV 23)
仆叁	*Pu Shen*	(Bl 61)	商阳	*Shang Yang*	(LI 1)
气冲	*Qi Chong*	(St 30)	膻中	*Shan Zhong*	(CV 17)
气海	*Qi Hai*	(CV 6)	少冲	*Shao Chong*	(Ht 9)
气海俞	*Qi Hai Shu*	(Bl 24)	少府	*Shao Fu*	(Ht 8)
气户	*Qi Hu*	(St 13)	少海	*Shao Hai*	(Ht 3)
瘛脉	*Qi Mai*	(TB 18)	少商	*Shao Shang*	(Lu 11)
期门	*Qi Men*	(Liv 14)	少泽	*Shao Ze*	(SI 1)
气舍	*Qi She*	(St 11)	神藏	*Shen Cang*	(Ki 25)
气穴	*Qi Xue*	(GB 40)	神道	*Shen Dao*	(GV 11)
前顶	*Qian Ding*	(GV 21)	神封	*Shen Feng*	(Ki 23)
强间	*Qiang Jian*	(GV 18)	申脉	*Shen Mai*	(Bl 62)
前谷	*Qian Gu*	(SI 2)	神门	*Shen Men*	(Ht 7)
窍阴	*Qiao Yin*	(GB 44 or GB 11)	神阙	*Shen Que*	(CV 8)
清冷渊	*Qing Leng Yuan*	(TB 11)	肾俞	*Shen Shu*	(Bl 23)
青灵	*Qing Ling*	(Ht 2)	神堂	*Shen Tang*	(Bl 44)
丘墟	*Qiu Xu*	(GB 40)	神庭	*Shen Ting*	(GV 24)
曲鬓	*Qu Bin*	(GB 7)	身柱	*Shen Zhu*	(GV 12)
曲差	*Qu Chai*	(Bl 4)	食窦	*Shi Dou*	(Sp 17)
曲池	*Qu Chi*	(LI 11)	石关	*Shi Guan*	(Ki 18)
曲骨	*Qu Gu*	(CV 2)	石门	*Shi Men*	(CV 5)
曲泉	*Qu Quan*	(Liv 8)	十宣	*Shi Xuan*	(M-UE-1)
曲垣	*Qu Yuan*	(SI 13)	手三里	*Shou San Li*	(LI 10)
曲泽	*Qu Ze*	(Per 3)	输府	*Shu Fu*	(Ki 27)
颧髎	*Quan Liao*	(SI 18)	束骨	*Shu Gu*	(Bl 65)
缺盆	*Que Pen*	(St 12)	率谷	*Shuai Gu*	(GB 8)
然谷	*Ran Gu*	(Ki 2)	水道	*Shui Dao*	(St 28)
人迎	*Ren Ying*	(St 9)	水分	*Shui Fen*	(CV 9)
人中	*Ren Zhong*	(GV 26)	水沟	*Shui Gou*	(GV 26)

水泉	*Shui Quan*	(Ki 5)		完骨	*Wan Gu*	(GB 12)
水突	*Shui Tu*	(St 10)		腕骨	*Wan Gu*	(SI 4)
四白	*Si Bai*	(St 2)		胃仓	*Wei Cang*	(Bl 50)
四渎	*Si Du*	(TB 9)		维道	*Wei Dao*	(GB 28)
四缝	*Si Feng*	(M-UE-9)		胃俞	*Wei Shu*	(Bl 21)
四满	*Si Man*	(Ki 14)		委阳	*Wei Yang*	(Bl 39)
四神聪	*Si Shen Cong*	(M-HN-1)		委中	*Wei Zhong*	(Bl 40)
丝竹空	*Si Zhu Kong*	(TB 23)		温溜	*Wen Liu*	(LI 7)
素髎	*Su Liao*	(GV 25)		五处	*Wu Chu*	(Bl 5)
太白	*Tai Bai*	(Sp 3)		五里	*Wu Li*	(Liv 10 & LI 13)
太坛	*Tai Chong*	(Liv 3)		五枢	*Wu Shu*	(GB 27)
太溪	*Tai Xi*	(Ki 3)		屋翳	*Wu Yi*	(St 15)
太阳	*Tai Yang*	(M-HN-9)		膝关	*Xi Guan*	(Liv 7)
太乙	*Tai Yi*	(St 23)		郄门	*Xi Men*	(Per 4)
太渊	*Tai Yuan*	(Lu 9)		膝眼	*Xi Yan*	(St 35)
陶道	*Tao Dao*	(GV 13)		膝阳关	*Xi Yang Guan*	(GB 33)
天池	*Tian Chi*	(Per 1)		下关	*Xia Guan*	(St 7)
天冲	*Tian Chong*	(GB 9)		下巨虚	*Xia Ju Xu*	(St 39)
天窗	*Tian Chuang*	(SI 16)		下廉	*Xia Lian*	(LI 8)
天鼎	*Tian Ding*	(LI 17)		下髎	*Xia Liao*	(Bl 34)
天府	*Tian Fu*	(Lu 3)		下脘	*Xia Wan*	(CV 10)
天井	*Tian Jing*	(TB 10)		侠溪	*Xia Xi*	(GB 43)
天髎	*Tian Liao*	(TB 15)		陷谷	*Xian Gu*	(St 43)
天泉	*Tian Quan*	(Per 2)		小肠俞	*Xiao Chang Shu*	(Bl 27)
天容	*Tian Rong*	(SI 17)		小海	*Xiao Hai*	(SI 8)
天枢	*Tian Shu*	(St 25)		消泺	*Xiao Luo*	(TB 12)
天突	*Tian Tu*	(CV 22)		囟会	*Xin Hui*	(GV 22)
天溪	*Tian Xi*	(Sp 18)		心俞	*Xin Shu*	(Bl 15)
天牖	*Tian You*	(TB 16)		行间	*Xing Jian*	(Liv 2)
天柱	*Tian Zhu*	(Bl 10)		胸乡	*Xiong Xiang*	(Sp 19)
天宗	*Tian Zong*	(SI 11)		璇玑	*Xuan Ji*	(CV 21)
条口	*Tiao Kou*	(St 38)		悬厘	*Xuan Li*	(GB 6)
听宫	*Ting Gong*	(SI 19)		悬颅	*Xuan Lu*	(GB 5)
听会	*Ting Hui*	(GB 2)		悬枢	*Xuan Shu*	(GV 5)
通谷	*Tong Gu*	(Bl 66)		悬钟	*Xuan Zhong*	(GB 39)
通里	*Tong Li*	(Ht 5)		血海	*Xue Hai*	(Sp 10)
通天	*Tong Tian*	(Bl 7)		哑门	*Ya Men*	(GV 15)
瞳子	*Tong Zi Liao*	(GB 1)		阳白	*Yang Bai*	(GB 14)
头临泣	*Tou Lin Qi*	(GB 15)		阳池	*Yang Chi*	(TB 4)
头维	*Tou Wei*	(St 8)		阳辅	*Yang Fu*	(GB 38)
外关	*Wai Guan*	(TB 5)		阳纲	*Yang Gang*	(Bl 48)
外陵	*Wai Ling*	(St 26)		阳谷	*Yang Gu*	(SI 5)
外丘	*Wai Qiu*	(GB 36)		阳交	*Yang Jiao*	(GB 35)

养老	*Yang Lao*	(SI 6)		支正	*Zhi Zheng*	(SI 7)
阳陵泉	*Yang Ling Quan*	(GB 34)		中冲	*Zhong Chong*	(Per 9)
阳溪	*Yang Xi*	(LI 5)		中渎	*Zhong Du*	(GB 32)
腰俞	*Yao Shu*	(GV 2)		中都	*Zhong Du*	(Liv 6)
腰眼	*Yao Yan*	(M-BW-24)		中封	*Zhong Feng*	(Liv 4)
腰阳关	*Yao Yang Guan*	(GV 3)		中府	*Zhong Fu*	(Lu 1)
液门	*Ye Men*	(TB 2)		中极	*Zhong Ji*	(CV 3)
翳风	*Yi Feng*	(TB 17)		中髎	*Zhong Liao*	(Bl 33)
意舍	*Yi She*	(Bl 49)		中俞	*Zhong Lu Shu*	(Bl 29)
譩譆	*Yi Xi*	(Bl 45)		中枢	*Zhong Shu*	(GV 7)
隐白	*Yin Bai*	(Sp 1)		中庭	*Zhong Ting*	(CV 16)
阴包	*Yin Bao*	(Liv 9)		中脘	*Zhong Wan*	(CV 12)
阴都	*Yin Du*	(Ki 19)		中渚	*Zhong Zhu*	(TB 3)
阴谷	*Yin Gu*	(Ki 10)		肘髎	*Zhou Liao*	(LI 12)
阴交	*Yin Jiao*	(GV 28)		周荣	*Zhou Rong*	(Sp 20)
阴廉	*Yin Lian*	(Liv 11)		筑宾	*Zhu Bin*	(Ki 9)
阴陵泉	*Yin Ling Quan*	(Sp 9)		足临泣	*Zu Lin Qi*	(GB 41)
殷门	*Yin Men*	(Bl 37)		足三里	*Zu San Li*	(St 36)
阴市	*Yin Shi*	(St 33)				
印堂	*Yin Tang*	(M-HN-3)				
阴郄	*Yin Xi*	(Ht 6)				
膺窗	*Ying Chuang*	(St 16)				
迎香	*Ying Xiang*	(LI 20)				
涌泉	*Yong Quan*	(Ki 1)				
幽门	*You Men*	(Ki 21)				
鱼际	*Yu Ji*	(Lu 10)				
玉堂	*Yu Tang*	(CV 18)				
鱼腰	*Yu Yao*	(M-HN-6)				
玉液	*Yu Ye*	(M-HN-20)				
玉枕	*Yu Zhen*	(Bl 9)				
彧中	*Yu Zhong*	(Ki 26)				
渊液	*Yuan Ye*	(GB 22)				
云门	*Yun Men*	(Lu 2)				
攒竹	*Zan Zhu*	(Bl 2)				
章门	*Zhang Men*	(Liv 13)				
照海	*Zhao Hai*	(Ki 6)				
辄筋	*Zhe Jin*	(GB 23)				
正营	*Zheng Ying*	(GB 17)				
秩边	*Zhi Bian*	(Bl 54)				
支沟	*Zhi Gou*	(TB 6)				
志室	*Zhi Shi*	(Bl 52)				
至阳	*Zhi Yang*	(GV 9)				
至阴	*Zhi Yin*	(Bl 67)				

Chinese medicinals

The following list of Chinese medicinals can be used in the same way. If you know you are translating a formula or other list of Chinese medicinal names, then look up the first character in the name. Once you have the Pinyin spelling, then scan down this list to find the second and, in some cases, third and fourth characters. It is a waste of time to look up both characters if you don't have to.

艾叶	*Ai Ye*	Folium Artemisiae Argyii
安息香	*An Xi Xiang*	Benzoinum
巴豆	*Ba Dou*	Semen Crotonis Tiglii
巴戟天	*Ba Ji Tian*	Radix Morindae Officinalis
八月札	*Ba Yue Zha*	Fructus Akebiae Trifoliatae
白扁豆	*Bai Bian Dou*	Semen Dolichoris Lablab
百部	*Bai Bu*	Radix Stemonae
白矾	*Bai Fan*	Alumen
白附子	*Bai Fu Zi*	Rhizoma Typhonii Gigantei
白果	*Bai Guo*	Semen Ginkgonis Bilobae
百合	*Bai He*	Bulbus Lilii
白化蛇	*Bai Hua She*	Agkistrodon Seu Bungarus
白芨	*Bai Ji*	Rhizoma Bletillae
白蒺藜	*Bai Ji Li*	Fructus Tribuli Terrestris
败酱草	*Bai Jiang Cao*	Herba Patriniae Heterophyllae Cum Radice
白芥子	*Bai Jie Zi*	Semen Sinapis Albae
白茅根	*Bai Mao Gen*	Rhizoma Imperatae Cylindricae
白前	*Bai Qian*	Radix Et Rhizoma Cynanchi Baiqian
白芍	*Bai Shao*	Radix Albus Paeoniae Lactiflorae
白术	*Bai Zhu*	Rhizoma Atractylodis Macrocephalae
白头翁	*Bai Tou Weng*	Radix Pulsatillae Chinensis
白薇	*Bai Wei*	Radix Cynanchi Atrati
白鲜皮	*Bai Xian Pi*	Cortex Radicis Dictamni Dasycarpi
白芷	*Bai Zhi*	Radix Angelicae Dahuricae
柏子仁	*Bai Zi Ren*	Semen Biotae Orientalis
半遍莲	*Ban Bian Lian*	Herba Lobeliae Chinensis Cum Radice
板蓝根	*Ban Lan Gen*	Radix Isatidis Seu Baphicacanthi
半夏	*Ban Xia*	Rhizoma Pinelliae Ternatae
半枝莲	*Ban Zhi Lian*	Radix Scutellariae Barbatae
北沙叁	*Bei Sha Shen*	Radix Glehniae Littoralis
扁蓄	*Bian Xu*	Herba Polygoni Avicularis
荜芨	*Bi Ba*	Fructus Piperis Longi
荜澄茄	*Bi Cheng Qie*	Fructus Litseae
蓖麻子	*Bi Ma Zi*	Semen Rici Communis
萆薢	*Bi Xie*	Rhizoma Dioscoreae Hypoglaucae

鳖甲	*Bie Jia*	Carapax Amydae Sinensis
槟榔	*Bin Lang*	Semen Arecae Catechu
冰片	*Bing Pian*	Borneolum
薄荷	*Bo He*	Herba Menthae Haplocalycis
补骨脂	*Bu Gu Zhi*	Fructus Psoraleae Corylifoliae
蚕沙	*Can Sha*	Excrementum Bombycis Mori
苍耳子	*Cang Er Zi*	Fructus Xanthii Siberici
苍术	*Cang Zhu*	Rhizoma Atractylodis
草豆蔻	*Cao Dou Kou*	Semen Alpiniae Katsumadai
草果	*Cao Guo*	Fructus Amomi Tsao-ko
侧柏叶	*Ce Bai Ye*	Cacumen Biotae Orientalis
柴胡	*Chai Hu*	Radix Bupleuri
蝉蜕	*Chan Tui*	Periostracum Cicadae
车前子	*Che Qian Zi*	Semen Plantaginis
陈皮	*Chen Pi*	Pericarpium Citri Reticulatae
陈棕炭	*Chen Zong Tan*	carbonized Stipula Trachycarpi
沉香	*Chen Xiang*	Lignum Aquilariae Agallochae
赤芍	*Chi Shao*	Radix Rubrus Paeoniae Lactiflorae
赤石脂	*Chi Shi Zhi*	Hallyositum Rubrum
赤小豆	*Chi Xiao Dou*	Semen Phaseoli Calcarati
茺蔚子	*Chong Wei Zi*	Semen Leonuri Heterophylli
楮根皮	*Chu Gen Pi*	Cortex Ailanthi Altissimae
川贝母	*Chuan Bei Mu*	Bulbus Fritillariae Cirrhosae
川椒	*Chuan Jiao*	Pericarpium Zanthoxyli Bungeani
穿山甲	*Chuan Shan Jia*	Squama Manitis Pentadactylis
川芎	*Chuan Xiong*	Radix Ligustici Wallichii
磁石	*Ci Shi*	Magnetitum
刺猬皮	*Ci Wei Pi*	Corium Erinacei
葱白	*Cong Bai*	Bulbus Allii Fistulosi
大腹皮	*Da Fu Pi*	Pericarpium Arecae Catechu
大簧	*Da Huang*	Radix Et Rhizoma Rhei
大蓟	*Da Ji*	Herba Cirsii Japonici
大戟	*Da Ji*	Radix Euphorbiae Seu Knoxiae
大青叶	*Da Qing Ye*	Folium Daqingye
大蒜	*Da Suan*	Bulbus Allii Sativi
大血藤	*Da Xue Teng*	Caulis Sargentodoxae
大枣	*Da Zao*	Fructus Zizyphi Jujubae
代赭石	*Dai Zhe Shi*	Haematitum
淡豆敊	*Dan Dou Chi*	Semen Praeparatum Sojae
胆南星	*Dan Nan Xing*	bile(-processed) Rhizoma Arisaematis
丹叁	*Dan Shen*	Radix Salviae Miltiorrhizae

淡竹叶	*Dan Zhu Ye*	Herba Lophatheri Gracilis
当归	*Dang Gui*	Radix Angelicae Sinensis
党参	*Dang Shen*	Radix Codonopsitis Pilosulae
灯心草	*Deng Xin Cao*	Medulla Junci Effusi
地肤子	*Di Fu Zi*	Fructus Kochiae Scopariae
地骨皮	*Di Gu Pi*	Cortex Radicis Lycii Chinensis
地黄	*Di Huang*	Radix Rehmanniae
地龙	*Di Long*	Lumbricus
地乳石	*Di Ru Shi*	Stalactitum
地榆	*Di Yu*	Radix Sanguisorbae
丁香	*Ding Xiang*	Flos Caryophylli
冬虫夏草	*Dong Chong Xia Cao*	Cordyceps Chinensis
冬瓜皮	*Dong Gua Pi*	Pericarpium Benincasae Hispidae
冬瓜子	*Dong Gua Zi*	Semen Benincasae Hispidae
冬葵子	*Dong Kui Zi*	Semen Abutilonis Seu Malvae
豆蔻	*Dou Kou*	Fructus Cardamomi
独活	*Du Huo*	Radix Angelicae Pubescentis
杜仲	*Du Zhong*	Cortex Eucommiae Ulmoidis
阿胶	*E Jiao*	Gelatinum Corii Asini
莪术	*E Zhu*	Rhizoma Curcumae Zedoariae
儿茶	*Er Cha*	Pasta Acaciae Seu Uncariae
番泻叶	*Fan Xie Ye*	Folium Sennae
防风	*Fang Feng*	Radix Ledebouriellae Divaricatae
防己	*Fang Ji*	Radix Stephaniae Tetrandrae
榧子	*Fei Zi*	Semen Torreyae Grandis
蜂房	*Feng Fang*	Nidus Vespae
佛手	*Fo Shou*	Fructus Citri Sacrodactylis
浮海石	*Fu Hai Shi*	Pumice
茯苓	*Fu Ling*	Sclerotium Poriae Cocos
茯苓皮	*Fu Ling Pi*	Cortex Sclerotii Poriae Cocos
伏龙肝	*Fu Long Gan*	Terra Flava Usta
覆盆子	*Fu Pen Zi*	Fructus Rubi Chingii
浮萍	*Fu Ping*	Herba Lemnae Seu Spirodelae
茯神	*Fu Shen*	Sclerotium Pararadicis Poriae Cocos
浮小麦	*Fu Xiao Mai*	Fructus Levis Tritici Aestivi
附子	*Fu Zi*	Radix Lateralis Praeparatus Aconiti Carmichaeli
甘草	*Gan Cao*	Radix Glycyrrhizae
干姜	*Gan Jiang*	dry Rhizoma Zingiberis
干漆	*Gan Qi*	Lacca Sinica Exsiccata
甘石	*Gan Shi*	Smithsonitum

甘松	*Gan Song*	Radix Et Rhizoma Nardostachydis
甘遂	*Gan Sui*	Radix Euphorbiae Kansui
藁本	*Gao Ben*	Radix Et Rhizoma Ligustici Chinensis
高良姜	*Gao Liang Jiang*	Rhizoma Alpiniae Officinari
葛根	*Ge Gen*	Radix Puerariae
蛤蚧	*Ge Jie*	Gecko
蛤壳	*Ge Ke*	Concha Cyclinae Sinensis
狗脊	*Gou Ji*	Rhizoma Cibotii Barometsis
枸杞子	*Gou Qi Zi*	Fructus Lycii Chinensis
钩藤	*Gou Teng*	Ramulus Uncariae Cum Uncis
谷草	*Gu Jing Cao*	Scapus Et Inflorescentia Eriocaulonis Buergeriani
骨碎补	*Gu Sui Bu*	Radix Drynariae
谷芽	*Gu Ya*	Fructus Germinatus Oryzae Sativae
栝楼	*Gua Lou*	Fructus Trichosanthis Kirlowii
栝楼皮	*Gua Lou Pi*	Pericarpium Trichosanthis Kirlowii
栝楼仁	*Gua Lou Ren*	Semen Trichosanthis Kirlowii
贯众	*Guan Zhong*	Rhizoma Guanchong
广防己	*Guang Fang Ji*	Radix Aristolochiae Fangchi
龟板	*Gui Ban*	Plastrum Testudinis
桂枝	*Gui Zhi*	Ramulus Cinnamomi Cassiae
海风藤	*Hai Feng Teng*	Caulis Piperis Futokadsurae
海蛤壳	*Hai Ge Ke*	Concha Cyclinae Sinensis
海金沙	*Hai Jin Sha*	Spora Lygodii Japonici
海螵蛸	*Hai Piao Xiao*	Os Sepiae Seu Sepiellae
海桐皮	*Hai Tong Pi*	Cortex Erythriniae
海乖	*Hai Zao*	Herba Sargassii
旱莲草	*Han Lian Cao*	Herba Ecliptae Prostratae
寒水石	*Han Shui Shi*	Calcitum
蒿本	*Hao Ben*	Radix Et Rhizoma Ligustici Chinensis
合换花	*He Huan Hua*	Flos Albizziae Julibrissinis
合欢皮	*He Huan Pi*	Cortex Albizziae Julibrissinis
何首乌	*He Shou Wu*	Radix Polygoni Multiflori
鹤虱	*He Shi*	Fructus Carpesii Seu Dauci
荷叶	*He Ye*	Folium Nelumbinis Nuciferae
荷子	*He Zi*	Fructus Terminaliae Chebulae
黑枣	*Hei Zao*	black Fructus Zizyphi Jujubae
黑芝麻	*Hei Zhi Ma*	black Semen Sesame Indici
红大戟	*Hong Da Ji*	Radix Euphorbiae Seu Knoxiae
红花	*Hong Hua*	Flos Carthami Tinctorii
红枣	*Hong Zao*	Fructus Zizyphi Jujubae
厚朴	*Hou Po*	Cortex Magnoliae Officinalis

虎骨	*Hu Gu*	Os Tigridis[1]
胡簧莲	*Hu Huang Lian*	Rhizoma Picrorrhizae
胡椒	*Hu Jiao*	Fructus Piperis Nigri
胡庐巴	*Hu Lu Ba*	Semen Trigonellae Foeni-graeci
胡麻仁	*Hu Ma Ren*	Semen Sesame Indici
琥魄	*Hu Po*	Succinum
胡桃仁	*Hu Tao Ren*	Semen Juglandis Regiae
掌杖	*Hu Zhang*	Radix Et Rhizoma Polygoni Cuspidati
花蕊石	*Hua Rui Shi*	Ophicalcitum
滑石	*Hua Shi*	Talcum
槐花米	*Huai Hua Mi*	Flos Immaturus Sophorae Japonicae
黄柏	*Huang Bai*	Cortex Phellodendri
黄丹	*Huang Dan*	Minium
黄精	*Huang Jing*	Rhizoma Polygonati
黄连	*Huang Lian*	Rhizoma Coptidis Chinensis
黄芪	*Huang Qi*	Radix Astragali Membranacei
黄芩	*Huang Qin*	Radix Scutellariae Baicalensis
火麻仁	*Huo Ma Ren*	Semen Cannabis Sativae
藿香	*Huo Xiang*	Herba Agastachis Seu Pogostemi
鸡内金	*Ji Nei Jin*	Endothelium Corneum Gigeriae Galli
鸡血藤	*Ji Xue Teng*	Caulis Milletiae Seu Spatholobi
姜黄	*Jiang Huang*	Rhizoma Curcumae Longae
降香	*Jiang Xiang*	Lignum Dalbergiae Odoriferae
桔梗	*Jie Geng*	Radix Platycodi Grandiflori
金千草	*Jin Qian Cao*	Herba Desmodii Styrachifolii
金樱子	*Jin Ying Zi*	Fructus Rosae Laevigatae
金银花	*Jin Yin Hua*	Flos Lonicerae Japonicae
荆芥	*Jing Jie*	Herba Seu Flos Schizonepetae Tenuifoliae
韭菜子	*Jiu Cai Zi*	Semen Allii Tuberosi
菊花	*Ju Hua*	Flos Chrysanthemi Morifolii
决明子	*Jue Ming Zi*	Semen Cassiae Torae
枯矾	*Ku Fan*	Alumen Praeparatum
苦楝皮	*Ku Lian Pi*	Cortex Radicis Meliae
苦叁	*Ku Shen*	Radix Sophorae Flavescentis
苦杏仁	*Ku Xing Ren*	Semen Pruni Armeniacae
款冬花	*Kuan Dong Hua*	Flos Tussilaginis Farfarae
昆布	*Kun Bu*	Thallus Algae

---

[1] Tiger bone is from a severely endangered species and should not be used in the manufacture of medicines. It can be replaced by Os Suis (*Zhu Gu*), pig bone.

莱菔子	*Lai Fu Zi*	Semen Raphani Sativi
雷丸	*Lei Wan*	Sclerotium Omphaliae Lapidescentis
藜芦	*Li Lu*	Radix Et Rhizoma Veratri
荔枝核	*Li Zhi He*	Semen Litchi Chinensis
连翘	*Lian Qiao*	Fructus Forsythiae Suspensae
连子	*Lian Zi*	Semen Nelumbinis Nuciferae
连子心	*Lian Zi Xin*	Plumula Nelumbinis Nuciferae
凌霄花	*Ling Xiao Hua*	Flos Campsitis
羚羊角	*Ling Yang Jiao*	Cornu Antelopis Saiga-tatarici[2]
刘寄	*Liu Ji Nu*	Herba Artemisiae Anomalae
龙齿	*Long Chi*	Dens Draconis
龙骨	*Long Gu*	Os Draconis
龙胆草	*Long Dan Cao*	Radix Gentianae Scabrae
漏芦	*Lou Lu*	Radix Rhapontici Seu Echinopsis
录豆	*Lu Dou*	Semen Phaseoli Munginis
根芦	*Lu Gen*	Rhizoma Phragmitis Communis
芦荟	*Lu Hui*	Herba Aloes
鹿角胶	*Lu Jiao Jiao*	Gelatinum Cornu Cervi
鹿角霜	*Lu Jiao Shuang*	Cornu Degelatinum Cervi
路路通	*Lu Lu Tong*	Fructus Liquidambaris Taiwaniae
鹿茸	*Lu Rong*	Cornu Parvum Cervi
络石藤	*Luo Shi Teng*	Caulis Trachelospermi Jasminoidis
马勃	*Ma Bo*	Fructificatio Lasiosphaerae Seu Calvatiae
马齿苋	*Ma Chi Xian*	Herba Portulacae Oleraceae
马兜铃	*Ma Dou Ling*	Fructus Aristolochiae
麻黄	*Ma Huang*	Herba Ephedrae
麻黄根	*Ma Huang Gen*	Radix Ephedrae
马钱子	*Ma Qian Zi*	Semen Strychnotis
麦门冬	*Mai Men Dong*	Tuber Ophiopogonis Japonici
麦芽	*Mai Ya*	Fructus Germinatus Hordei Vulgaris
蔓荆子	*Man Jing Zi*	Fructus Viticis
芒硝	*Mang Xiao*	Mirabilitum
密蒙花	*Mi Meng Hua*	Flos Buddleiae
蜜陀僧	*Mi Tuo Seng*	Lithargyrum
明矾	*Ming Fan*	Alumen
没药	*Mo Yao*	Resina Myrrhae
牡丹皮	*Mu Dan Pi*	Cortex Radicis Moutan
木瓜	*Mu Gua*	Fructus Chaenomelis Lagenariae
牡蛎	*Mu Li*	Concha Ostreae

---

[2] Saiga antelope is an endangered species and its horn should not be used in the manufacture of medicine. It can be replaced by Cornu Caprae (*Shan Yang Jiao*), goat horn.

木通	*Mu Tong*	Caulis Akebiae
木香	*Mu Xiang*	Radix Auklandiae Lappae
木贼	*Mu Zei*	Herba Equiseti Hiemalis
南瓜子	*Nan Gua Zi*	Semen Cucurbitae Moschatae
牛旁子	*Niu Bang Zi*	Fructus Arctii Lappae
牛黄	*Niu Huang*	Calculus Bovis
牛膝	*Niu Xi*	Radix Achyranthis Bidentatae
女真子	*Nu Zhen Zi*	Fructus Ligustri Lucidi
藕节	*Ou Jie*	Nodus Rhizomatis Nelumbinis Nuciferae
胖大海	*Pang Da Hai*	Fructus Sterculiae Scaphageriae
炮姜	*Pao Jiang*	blast-fried Rhizoma Zingiberis
佩兰	*Pei Lan*	Herba Eupatorii Fortunei
硼砂	*Peng Sha*	Borax
枇杷叶	*Pi Pa Ye*	Folium Eriobotryae Japonicae
蒲公英	*Pu Gong Ying*	Herba Taraxaci Mongolici Cum Radice
蒲黄	*Pu Huang*	Pollen Typhae
茜草	*Qian Cao*	Radix Rubiae Cordifoliae
前胡	*Qian Hu*	Radix Peucedani
牵牛子	*Qian Niu Zi*	Semen Pharbiditis
芡实	*Qian Shi*	Semen Euryalis Ferocis
羌活	*Qiang Huo*	Radix Et Rhizoma Notopterygii
秦艽	*Qin Jiao*	Radix Gentianae Macrophyllae
秦皮	*Qin Pi*	Cortex Fraxini
青蒿	*Qing Hao*	Herba Artemisiae Apiaceae
青礞石	*Qing Meng Shi*	Lapis Chloriti
青皮	*Qing Pi*	Pericarpium Citri Reticulatae Viride
青葙子	*Qing Xiang Zi*	Semen Celosiae Argentae
瞿麦	*Qu Mai*	Herba Dianthi
全蝎	*Quan Xie*	Buthus Martensis
忍冬藤	*Ren Dong Teng*	Caulis Lonicerae Japonicae
人叁	*Ren Shen*	Radix Panacis Ginseng
肉苁蓉	*Rou Cong Rong*	Herba Cistanchis Deserticolae
肉豆蔻	*Rou Dou Kou*	Semen Myristicae Fragrantis
肉桂	*Rou Gui*	Cortex Cinnamomi Cassiae
乳香	*Ru Xiang*	Resina Olibani
三棱	*San Leng*	Rhizoma Sparganii
三七	*San Qi*	Radix Pseudoginseng

桑白皮	*Sang Bai Pi*	Cortex Radicis Mori Albi
桑寄生	*Sang Ji Sheng*	Ramulus Loranthi Seu Visci
桑螵蛸	*Sang Piao Xiao*	Ootheca Mantidis
桑葚	*Sang Shen*	Fructus Mori Albi
桑叶	*Sang Ye*	Folium Mori Albi
桑枝	*Sang Zhi*	Ramulus Mori Albi
砂仁	*Sha Ren*	Fructus Amomi
沙苑子	*Sha Yuan Zi*	Semen Astragali Complanati
山茨菇	*Shan Ci Gu*	Pseudobulbus Shancigu
山豆根	*Shan Dou Gen*	Radix Sophorae Subprostratae
山药	*Shan Yao*	Radix Dioscoreae Oppositae
山楂	*Shan Zha*	Fructus Crataegi
山茱萸	*Shan Zhu Yu*	Fructus Corni Officinalis
商陆	*Shang Lu*	Radix Phytolaccae
蛇床子	*She Chuang Zi*	Fructus Cnidii Monnieri
射干	*She Gan*	Rhizoma Belamcandae
蛇蜕	*She Tui*	Exuvia Serpentis
麝香	*She Xiang*	Secretio Moschi Moschiferi
神曲	*Shen Qu*	Massa Medica Fermentata
升麻	*Sheng Ma*	Rhizoma Cimicifugae
生姜	*Sheng Jiang*	uncooked Rhizoma Zingiberis
生铁落	*Sheng Tie Luo*	Frusta Ferri
石菖蒲	*Shi Chang Pu*	Rhizoma Acori Graminei
柿蒂	*Shi Di*	Calyx Khaki
石膏	*Shi Gao*	Gypsum Fibrosum
石斛	*Shi Hu*	Herba Dendrobii
石决明	*Shi Jue Ming*	Concha Haliotidis
使君子	*Shi Jun Zi*	Fructus Quisqualis
石榴皮	*Shi Liu Pi*	Pericarpium Punicae Granati
石苇	*Shi Wei*	Herba Pyrrosiae
首乌藤	*Shou Wu Teng*	Caulis Polygoni Multiflori
熟地黄	*Shu Di Huang*	cooked Radix Rehmanniae
水蛭	*Shui Zhi*	Hirudo
苏合香	*Su He Xiang*	Styrax Liquidis
苏木	*Su Mu*	Lignum Sappan
酸枣仁	*Suan Zao Ren*	Semen Zizyphi Spinosae
锁阳	*Suo Yang*	Herba Cynomorii Songarici
太子参	*Tai Zi Shen*	Radix Pseudostellariae
檀香	*Tan Xiang*	Lignum Santali Albi
桃仁	*Tao Ren*	Semen Pruni Persicae
天分	*Tian Hua Fen*	Radix Trichosanthis Kirlowii
天麻	*Tian Ma*	Rhizoma Gastrodiae

天门冬	*Tian Men Dong*	Tuber Asparagi Cochinensis
天南星	*Tian Nan Xing*	Rhizoma Arisaematis
天竺黄	*Tian Zhu Huang*	Concretio Silicea Bambusae
葶苈子	*Ting Li Zi*	Semen Descurainiae Seu Lepidii
通草	*Tong Cao*	Medulla Tetrapanacis Papyriferi
土鳖虫	*Tu Bie Chong*	Eupolyphaga Seu Opistholpatia
土茯苓	*Tu Fu Ling*	Rhizoma Smilacis Galbrae
菟丝子	*Tu Si Zi*	Semen Cuscutae Chinensis
瓦楞子	*Wa Leng Zi*	Concha Arcae Inflatae
王不留行	*Wang Bu Liu Xing*	Semen Vaccariae Segetalis
苇茎	*Wei Jing*	Rhizoma Phragmitis Communis
威灵仙	*Wei Ling Xian*	Radix Clematidis Chinensis
五倍子	*Wu Bei Zi*	Galla Rhois
蜈蚣	*Wu Gong*	Scolopendra Subspinipes
五加皮	*Wu Jia Pi*	Cortex Radicis Acanthopanacis Gracistyli
五灵脂	*Wu Ling Zhi*	Feces Trogopterori Seu Pteromi
乌梅	*Wu Mei*	Fructus Pruni Mume
乌梢蛇	*Wu Shao She*	Zaocys Dhumnades
五味子	*Wu Wei Zi*	Fructus Schisandrae Chinensis
乌药	*Wu Yao*	Radix Linderae Strychnifoliae
乌贼骨	*Wu Zei Gu*	Os Sepiae Sepiellae
吴茱萸	*Wu Zhu Yu*	Fructus Evodiae Rutaecarpae
西瓜	*Xi Gua*	Fructus Citrulli Vulgaris
犀角	*Xi Jiao*	Cornu Rhinocerotis[3]
豨莶草	*Xi Xian Cao*	Herba Siegesbeckiae
细辛	*Xi Xin*	Herba Asari Cum Radice
西洋叁	*Xi Yang Shen*	Radix Panacis Qinquifolii
夏枯草	*Xia Ku Cao*	Spica Prunellae Vulgaris
仙鹤草	*Xian He Cao*	Herba Agrimoniae Pilosae
仙灵脾	*Xian Ling Pi*	Herba Epimedii
仙茅	*Xian Mao*	Rhizoma Curculiginis Orchioidis
香附	*Xiang Fu*	Rhizoma Cyperi Rotundi
香薷	*Xiang Ru*	Herba Elsholtziae
小茴囤	*Xiao Hui Xiang*	Fructus Foeniculi Vulgaris
薤白	*Xie Bai*	Bulbus Allii
辛夷	*Xin Yi*	Flos Magnoliae Lilliflorae
杏仁	*Xing Ren*	Semen Pruni Armeniacae
熊胆	*Xiong Dan*	Fel Ursi[3]

---

[3] Rhinoceri and bears are endangered species and neither rhino horn nor bear gall should not be used in the manufacture of medicines.

雄黄	*Xiong Huang*	Realgar
续断	*Xu Duan*	Radix Dipsaci
旋覆花	*Xuan Fu Hua*	Flos Inulae
玄参	*Xuan Shen*	Radix Scrophulariae Ningpoensis
血竭	*Xue Jie*	Sanguis Draconis
血余炭	*Xue Yu Tan*	Crinis Carbonisatus
鸦蛋子	*Ya Dan Zi*	Fructus Bruceae Javanicae
延胡索	*Yan Hu Suo*	Rhizoma Corydalis Yanhusuo
阳起石	*Yang Qi Shi*	Actinolitum
野菊花	*Ye Ju Hua*	Flos Chrysanthemi Indici
益母草	*Yi Mu Cao*	Herba Leonuri Heterophylli
饴糖	*Yi Tang*	Saccharum Granorum
薏苡仁	*Yi Yi Ren*	Semen Coicis Lachyrma-jobi
益知仁	*Yi Zhi Ren*	Fructus Alpiniae Oxyphyllae
阴柴胡	*Yin Chai Hu*	Radix Stellariae Dichotomae
茵陈	*Yin Chen*	Herba Artemisiae Capillaris
阴阳藿	*Yin Yang Huo*	Herba Epimedii
罂粟壳	*Ying Su Ke*	Pericarpium Papaveris Somniferi
由松结	*You Song Jie*	Nodus Ligni Pini
郁金	*Yu Jin*	Tuber Curcumae
郁李仁	*Yu Li Ren*	Semen Pruni
禹馀粮	*Yu Yu Liang*	Limonitum
鱼腥草	*Yu Xing Cao*	Herba Houttuyniae Cordatae Cum Radice
玉竹	*Yu Zhu*	Rhizoma Polygonati Odorati
芫花	*Yuan Hua*	Flos Daphnis Genkwae
元志	*Yuan Zhi*	Radix Polygalae Tenuifoliae
元参	*Yuan Shen*	Radix Scrophulariae Ningpoensis
月季花	*Yue Ji Hua*	Flos Et Fructus Rosae Chinensis
藏红花	*Zang Hong Hua*	Stigma Croci Sativi
皂角刺	*Zao Jiao Ci*	Spina Gleditschiae Sinensis
泽兰	*Ze Lan*	Herba Lycopi Lucidi
泽泻	*Ze Xie*	Rhizoma Alismatis
章脑	*Zhang Nao*	Camphora
浙贝母	*Zhe Bei Mu*	Bulbus Fritillariae Thunbergii
珍珠	*Zhen Zhu*	Margarita
珍珠母	*Zhen Zhu Mu*	Concha Margaratiferae
枳壳	*Zhi Ke*	Fructus Citri Aurantii
知母	*Zhi Mu*	Rhizoma Anemarrhenae Aspheloidis
枳实	*Zhi Shi*	Fructus Immaturus Citri Aurantii
栀子	*Zhi Zi*	Fructus Gardeniae Jasminoidis
竹沥	*Zhu Li*	Succus Bambusae

猪苓	*Zhu Ling*	Sclerotium Polypori Umbellati
竹茹	*Zhu Ru*	Caulis Bambusae In Taeniis
朱砂	*Zhu Sha*	Cinnabar
紫草	*Zi Cao*	Radix Lithospermi Seu Arnebiae
紫河车	*Zi He Che*	Placenta Hominis
紫花地丁	*Zi Hua Di Ding*	Herba Violae Yedoensitis Cum Radice
自然铜	*Zi Ran Tong*	Pyritum
紫石英	*Zi Shi Ying*	Fluoritum
紫苏根	*Zi Su Gen*	Caulis Perillae Frutescentis
紫苏叶	*Zi Su Ye*	Folium Perillae Frutescentis
紫苏子	*Zi Su Zi*	Fructus Perillae Frutescentis
紫菀	*Zi Wan*	Radix Asteris Tatarici

Medicinal formula names

The following list of approximately 90 Chinese medicinal formula names is taken from *Seventy Essential TCM Formulas*. This is a repertoire of the 90 standard formulas taught at the provincial Chinese medical colleges in the People's Republic of China. There are hundreds and thousands of other Chinese formulas, but these are some of the most famous and commonly used ones. Again, to use this cheat sheet, look up the first character of a formula and then scan the Pinyin list for a match with the rest of the characters in the name. Then make sure that all the Chinese characters match.

艾附暖宫丸	*Ai Fu Nuan Gong Wan*	Mugwort & Cyperus Warm the Uterus Pills
安宫牛黄丸	*An Gong Niu Huang Wan*	Quiet the Palace Bezoar Pills
八味地黄丸	*Ba Wei Di Huang Wan*	Eight Flavors Rehmannia Pills
八仙长寿丸	*Ba Xian Chang Shou Wan*	Eight Immortals Long Life Pills
八珍汤	*Ba Zhen Tang*	Eight Pearls Pills
八正汤	*Ba Zheng Tang*	Eight (Ingredients) Correcting Decoction
败毒散	*Bai Du San*	Vanquish Toxins Powder
百合固金汤	*Bai He Gu Jin Tang*	Lily Secure Metal Decoction
白虎汤	*Bai Hu Tang*	White Tiger Decoction
白头翁汤	*Bai Tou Weng Tang*	Pulsatilla Decoction
半夏白术天麻汤 *Ban Xia Bai Zhu Tian Ma Tang*		Pinellia, Atractylodes & Gastrodia Decoction
半夏泻心汤	*Ban Xia Xie Xin Tang*	Pinellia Drain the Heart Decoction
保和丸	*Bao He Wan*	Protect Harmony Pills
贝母栝楼散	*Bei Mu Gua Lou San*	Fritillaria & Trichosanthes Powder
补中益气汤	*Bu Zhong Yi Qi Tang*	Supplement the Center & Boost the Qi Decoction
柴胡桂枝汤	*Chai Hu Gui Zhi Tang*	Bupleurum & Cinnamon Twig Decoction

柴胡龙骨牡蛎汤
    Chai Hu Long Gu Mu Li Tang Bupleurum, Dragon Bone & Oyster Shell Decoction

大柴胡汤	*Da Chai Hu Tang*	Major Bupleurum Decoction
大承气汤	*Da Cheng Qi Tang*	Major Order the Qi Decoction
大青龙汤	*Da Qing Long Tang*	Major Blue-green Dragon Decoction
丹栀逍遥散	*Dan Zhi Xiao Yao San*	Moutan & Gardenia Rambling Powder
当归六黄汤	*Dang Gui Liu Huang Tang*	Dang Gui Six Yellows Decoction
当归芍药散	*Dang Gui Shao Yao San*	Dang Gui & Peony Powder
导赤散	*Dao Chi San*	Abduct the Red Powder
导痰汤	*Dao Tan Tang*	Abduct Phlegm Decoction
独活寄生汤	*Du Huo Ji Sheng Tang*	Angelica Pubescens & Loranthus Decoction
气丸	*Du Qi Wan*	Capital Qi Pills

二陈汤	*Er Chen Tang*	Two Aged (Ingredients) Decoction
二妙散	*Er Miao San*	Two Wonders Powder
二仙汤	*Er Xian Tang*	Two Immortals Decoction

甘草泻心汤	*Gan Cao Xie Xin Tang*	Licorice Drain the Heart Decoction
隔下逐瘀汤	*Ge Xia Zhu Yu Tang*	Below the Diaphragm Dispel Stasis Decoction
归脾汤	*Gui Pi Tang*	Restore the Spleen Decoction

桂枝加龙骨牡蛎汤
    Gui Zhi Jia Long Gu Mu Li Tang
    Cinnamon Twig, Dragon Bone & Oyster Shell Decoction

桂枝汤	*Gui Zhi Tang*	Cinnamon Twig Decoction

黄连解毒烫	*Huang Lian Jie Du Tang*	Coptis Resolve Toxins Decoction
黄连温胆汤	*Huang Lian Wen Dan Tang*	Coptis Warm the Gallbladder Decoction

胶艾汤	*Jiao Ai Tang*	Donkey Skin Glue & Mugwort Decoction
金匮肾气丸	*Jin Gui Shen Qi Wan*	Golden Cabinet Kidney Qi Pills
橘皮竹茹汤	*Ju Pi Zhu Ru Tang*	Orange Peel & Caulis Bambusae Decoction

苓桂术甘汤	*Ling Gui Zhu Gan Tang*	Poria, Cinnamon, Atractylodes & Licorice Decoction
六君子汤	*Liu Jun Zi Tang*	Six Gentlemen Decoction
六味地黄丸	*Liu Wei Di Huang Wan*	Six Flavors Rehmannia Pills
六一散	*Liu Yi San*	Six to One Powder
龙胆泻肝汤	*Long Dan Xie Gan Tang*	Gentiana Drain the Liver Decoction

麻黄汤	*Ma Huang Tang*	Ephedra Decoction

麻杏甘石汤	*Ma Xing Gan Shi Tang*	Ephedra, Armeniaca, Licorice & Gypsum Decoction
麻子仁丸	*Ma Zi Ren Wan*	Cannabis Pills
明目地黄丸	*Ming Mu Di Huang Wan*	Brighten the Eyes Rehmannia Pills
平胃散	*Ping Wei San*	Level the Stomach Powder
杞菊地黄丸	*Qi Ju Di Huang Wan*	Lycium & Chrysanthemum Rehmannia Pills
芩连四物汤	*Qin Lian Si Wu Tang*	Scutellaria & Coptis Four Materials Decoction
青蒿鳖甲汤	*Qing Hao Bie Jia Tang*	Artemisia Capillaris & Carapax Amydae Decoction
清气化痰丸	*Qing Qi Hua Tan Wan*	Clear the Qi & Transform Phlegm Pills
人参白虎汤	*Ren Shen Bai Hu Tang*	Ginseng White Tiger Decoction
三拗汤	*San Ao Tang*	Three Rough & Ready (Ingredients) Decoction
三妙散	*San Miao San*	Three Wonders Powder
桑菊饮	*Sang Ju Yin*	Morus & Chrysanthemum Drink
桑螵蛸散	*Sang Piao Xiao San*	Mantis Eggcase Powder
少腹逐瘀汤	*Shao Fu Zhu Yu Tang*	Lower Abdomen Dispel Stasis Decoction
参苓白术散	*Shen Ling Bai Zhu San*	Ginseng, Poria & Atractylodes Powder
生化汤	*Sheng Hua Tang*	Engendering & Transforming Decoction
生姜泻心汤	*Sheng Jiang Xie Xin Tang*	Uncooked Ginger Drain the Heart Decoction
圣愈汤	*Sheng Yu Tang*	Sagely Curing Decoction
十灰散	*Shi Hui San*	Ten Ashes Powder
十全大补汤	*Shi Quan Da Bu Tang*	Ten (Ingredients) Greatly & Completely Supplementing Decoction
失笑散	*Shi Xiao San*	Loose a Smile Powder
十枣汤	*Shi Zao Tang*	Ten Dates Decoction
四君子汤	*Si Jun Zi Tang*	Four Gentlemen Decoction
四妙散	*Si Miao San*	Four Wonders Powder
四逆散	*Si Ni San*	Four Counterflows Powder
四逆汤	*Si Ni Tang*	Four Counterflows Decoction
四神丸	*Si Shen Wan*	Four Spirits Pills
四物汤	*Si Wu Tang*	Four Materials Decoction
酸枣仁汤	*Suan Zao Ren Tang*	Zizyphus Spinosa Decoction
桃红四物汤	*Tao Hong Si Wu Tang*	Persica & Carthamus Four Materials Decoction
天麻钩藤饮	*Tian Ma Gou Teng Yin*	Gastrodia & Uncaria Drink
调胃承气汤	*Tiao Wei Cheng Qi Tang*	Regulate the Stomach & Order the Qi Decoction
调中益气汤	*Tiao Zhong Yi Qi Tang*	Regulate the Center & Boost the Qi Decoction
完带汤	*Wan Dai Tang*	End Vaginal Discharge Decoction
胃苓散	*Wei Ling San*	Stomach(-quieting) Poria Decoction

温胆汤	*Wen Dan Tang*	Warm the Gallbladder Decoction
温清饮	*Wen Qing Yin*	Warming & Clearing Drink
五苓散	*Wu Ling San*	Five (Ingredients) Poria Powder
乌梅丸	*Wu Mei Wan*	Mume Pills
犀角地黄汤	*Xi Jiao Di Huang Tang*	Rhinoceros Horn & Rehmannia Decoction
香砂六君子汤	*Xiang Sha Liu Jun Zi Tang*	Auklandia & Amomum Six Gentlemen Decoction
小柴胡汤	*Xiao Chai Hu Tang*	Minor Bupleurum Decoction
小承气汤	*Xiao Cheng Qi Tang*	Minor Order the Qi Decoction
小青龙汤	*Xiao Qing Long Tang*	Minor Blue-green Dragon Decoction
逍遥散	*Xiao Yao San*	Rambling Powder
血府逐瘀汤	*Xue Fu Zhu Yu Tang*	Blood Chamber Dispel Stasis Decoction
阴陈蒿汤	*Yin Chen Hao Tang*	Artemisia Capillaris Decoction
阴陈五苓散	*Yin Chen Wu Ling San*	Artemisia Capillaris Five (Ingredients) Poria Powder
银翘散	*Yin Qiao San*	Lonicera & Forsythia Powder
越鞠丸	*Yue Ju Wan*	Escape Restraint Pills
增液承气汤	*Zeng Ye Cheng Qi Tang*	Increase Humors & Order the Qi Decoction
镇肝熄风汤	*Zhen Gan Xi Feng Tang*	Settle the Liver & Extinguish Wind Decoction
知白地黄丸	*Zhi Bai Di Huang Wan*	Anemarrhena & Phellodendron Rehmannia Pills
朱砂安神丸	*Zhu Sha An Shen Wan*	Cinnabar Quiet the Spirit Pills
佐金丸	*Zuo Jin Wan*	Left Metal Pills

Famous Chinese Medical Book Titles

It is not uncommon to come across the names of famous Chinese books quoted in other books or cited or quoted in Chinese journal articles. These titles are usually given in quotation marks (" ") or double chevrons (《 》). Below is a list of some commonly occurring Chinese medical titles. If you think you are dealing with such a book title, look up the first character and then scan the list below to see if you can match the rest of the characters.

内经	*Nei Jing, Inner Classic*
素问	*Su Wen, Simple Questions*
灵枢	*Ling Shu, Spiritual Axis*
难经	*Nan Jing, Classic of Difficulties*
伤寒论	*Shang Han Lun, Treatise on Damage [Due to] Cold*
金匮要略	*Jin Gui Yao Lue, Essentials from the Golden Cabinet*
甲乙经	*Jia Yi Jing, The Systematic Classic*
类经	*Lei Jing, The Categorized Classic*
神农本草	*Shen Nong Ben Cao, The Divine Farmer's Materia Medica*

本草纲目	*Ben Cao Gang Mu, The Great Outline of Materia Medica*
脉经	*Mai Jing, The Pulse Classic*
濒湖脉学	*Bin Hu Mai Xue, The Lakeside Master's Study of the Pulse*
针灸大成	*Zhen Jiu Da Cheng, The Great Compendium of Acupuncture & Moxibustion*
景岳全书	*Jing Yue Quan Shu, [Zhang] Jing-yue's Complete Book*
傅青主女科	*Fu Qing Zhu Nu Ke, Fu Qing-zhu's Gynecology*
脾胃论	*Pi Wei Lun, Treatise on the Spleen & Stomach*
丹溪心法	*Dan Xi Xin Fa, [Zhu] Dan-xi's Heart Methods*
诸病原候论	*Zhu Bing Yuan Hou Lun, Treatise on the Causes & Symptoms of Diseases*

Pattern names

The following list of pattern names is yet another aid to help you get started with a minimum of effort. As with the other "cheat sheets" above, if you know that you are dealing with a pattern name, look up the first character in your Chinese-English dictionary and then scan the alphabetized Pinyin list to match up the other characters. This list is not definitively complete. There is a great deal of latitude and personal preference in the naming of patterns. However, it should help you get started. Just studying this list of pattern names will probably increase your understanding of TCM patterns.

表寒里热	*biao han li re*	exterior cold, interior heat
表热里寒	*biao re li han*	exterior heat, interior cold
冲任不补	*chong ren bu gu*	*chong* & *ren* not securing
冲任不调	*chong ren bu tiao*	*chong* & *ren* not regulated
冲任失调	*chong ren shi tiao*	loss of regulation of the *chong* & *ren*
冲任损伤	*chong ren sun shang*	*chong* & *ren* detriment and damage
大肠寒结	*da chang han jie*	large intestine cold binding
大肠湿热	*da chang shi re*	large intestine damp heat
大肠虚	*da chang xu*	large intestine vacuity
大肠虚寒	*da chang xu han*	large intestine vacuity cold
大肠液亏	*da chang ye kui*	large intestine humor depletion
胆热	*dan re*	gallbladder heat
胆实	*dan shi*	gallbladder repletion
胆虚	*dan xu*	gallbladder vacuity
肺火	*fei huo*	lung fire
肺津不布	*fei jin bu bu*	lung fluids not distributed
肺络损伤	*fei luo sun shang*	lung network vessel detriment & damage
肺气不利	*fei qi bu li*	inhibition of the lung qi
肺气不宣	*fei qi bu xuan*	lung qi not diffusing
肺气虚	*fei qi xu*	lung qi vacuity

肺热	*fei re*	lung heat
肺肾两虚	*fei shen liang xu*	lung-kidney dual vacuity
肺肾气虚	*fei shen qi xu*	lung-kidney qi vacuity
肺肾阴虚	*fei shen yin xu*	lung-kidney yin vacuity
肺实	*fei shi*	lung repletion
肺失清肃	*fei shi qing su*	lung loss of clearing & depurating
肺虚	*fei xu*	lung vacuity
肺阴虚	*fei yin xu*	lung yin vacuity
肺阴虚燥	*fei yin xu zao*	lung yin vacuity dryness
肺燥	*fei zao*	lung dryness
伏热在里	*fu re zai li*	deep-lying heat in the interior
肝胆气虚	*gan dan qi xu*	liver-gallbladder qi vacuity
肝胆湿热	*gan dan shi re*	liver-gallbladder damp heat
肝凤内动	*gan feng nei dong*	liver wind stirring internally
肝寒	*gan han*	liver cold
肝火	*gan huo*	liver fire
肝火上炎	*gan huo shang yan*	liver fire flaring upward
肝气犯脾	*gan qi fan pi*	liver qi assails the spleen
肝气犯胃	*gan qi fan wei*	liver qi assails the stomach
肝气上逆	*gan qi shang ni*	liver qi counterflowing upward
肝热	*gan re*	liver fire
肝肾亏损	*gan shen kui sun*	liver-kidney depletion & detriment
肝肾两虚	*gan shen liang xu*	liver-kidney dual vacuity
肝血虚	*gan xue xu*	liver blood vacuity
肝阳上亢	*gan yang shang kang*	ascendant hyperactivity of liver yang
肝阴虚	*gan yin xu*	liver yin vacuity
肝郁脾虚	*gan yu pi xu*	liver depression, spleen vacuity
肝郁气滞	*gan yu qi zhi*	liver depression qi stagnation
寒极生热	*han ji sheng re*	extreme cold engenders heat
寒凝肝脉	*han ning gan mai*	cold congelation in the liver vessel
寒凝气滞	*han ning qi zhi*	cold congelation qi stagnation
寒痰阻肺	*han tan zu fei*	cold phlegm obstructing the lungs
久热伤阴	*jiu re shang yin*	enduring heat damages yin
龙火内燔	*long huo nei fan*	dragon fire internally blazing
命门火旺	*ming men huo wang*	life gate fire effulgence
膀胱气闭	*pang guang qi bi*	bladder qi block
膀胱湿热	*pang guang shi re*	bladder damp heat

膀胱虚寒	*pang guang xu han*	bladder vacuity cold
脬气不固	*pao qi bu gu*	bladder qi not securing
脾不统血	*pi bu tong xue*	spleen not managing (*i.e.*, restraining) the blood
脾肺两虚	*pi fei liang xu*	spleen-lung dual vacuity
脾气不升	*pi qi bu sheng*	spleen qi not upbearing
脾气虚	*pi qi xu*	spleen qi vacuity
脾热	*pi re*	spleen heat
脾肾阳虚	*pi shen yang xu*	spleen-kidney yang vacuity
脾失健运	*pi shi jian yun*	spleen loss of fortification & movement
脾失运化	*pi shi yun hua*	spleen loss of movement & transformation
脾胃湿热	*pi wei shi re*	spleen-stomach damp heat
脾胃虚弱	*pi wei xu ruo*	spleen-stomach vacuity weakness
脾虚	*pi xu*	spleen vacuity
脾虚湿困	*pi xu shi kun*	spleen vacuity, damp encumbrance
脾阳虚	*pi yang xu*	spleen yang vacuity
脾阴虚	*pi yin xu*	spleen yin vacuity
气化不利	*qi hua bu li*	inhibition of qi transformation
气机不利	*qi ji bu li*	inhibition of the qi mechanism
气隧血脱	*qi sui xue tuo*	qi follows blood desertion
气虚中满	*qi xu zhong man*	qi vacuity central fullness
气血两虚	*qi xue liang xu*	qi & blood dual vacuity
气血失调	*qi xue shi tiao*	qi & blood loss of regulation
气阴两虚	*qi yin liang xu*	qi & yin dual vacuity
气滞血瘀	*qi zhi xue yu*	qi stagnation & blood stasis
热伏冲任	*re fu chong ren*	heat deep-lying or hidden in the *chong & ren*
热极生寒	*re ji sheng han*	extreme heat engenders cold
热结膀胱	*re jie pang guang*	heat bound in the bladder
热结下蕉	*re jie xia jiao*	heat bound in the lower burner
热入心包	*re ru xin bao*	heat entering the pericardium
热入血分	*re ru xue fen*	heat entering the blood phase
热入血室	*re ru xue shi*	heat entering the blood chamber
热伤肺络	*re shang fei luo*	heat damaging the lung network vessels
热伤筋脉	*re shang jin mai*	heat damaging the sinews and vessels (or sinew vessels)
热伤神明	*re shang shen ming*	heat damaging the spirit brightness
热盛气分	*re sheng qi fen*	heat exuberance in the qi division
热邪阻肺	*re xie zu fei*	heat evils obstructing the lungs
热灼肾阴	*re zhuo shen yin*	heat burning kidney yin
三蕉湿热	*san jiao shi re*	triple burner damp heat
三蕉虚寒	*san jiao xu han*	triple burner vacuity cold
上寒下热	*shang han xia re*	above cold, below heat

上热下寒	*shang re xia han*	above heat, below cold
伤损及下	*shang sun ji xia*	detriment above reaching below
少阴寒化	*shao yin han hua*	*shao yin* cold transformation
少阴热化	*shao yin re hua*	*shao yin* heat transformation
肾气不固	*shen qi bu gu*	kidney qi not securing
肾虚	*shen xu*	kidney vacuity
肾溆水泛	*shen xu shui fan*	kidney vacuity, water flooding
肾阳虚	*sheng yang xu*	kidney yang vacuity
肾阳虚衰	*shen yang xu shuai*	kidney yang vacuity and debility
肾阴虚	*shen yin xu*	kidney yin vacuity
升降失常	*sheng jiang shi chang*	upbearing & downbearing lose their normalcy
湿热内熏	*shi re nei xun*	dampness & heat internally brewing
湿热下蕉	*shi re xia jiao*	damp heat in the lower burner
湿热瘀滞	*shi re yu zhi*	damp heat stasis & stagnation
湿胜阳微	*shi sheng yang wei*	dampness prevailing, yang becoming slight
湿郁热伏	*shi yu re fu*	damp depression, heat deeply lying
食滞胃腕	*shi zhi wei wan*	food stagnating in the stomach venter
湿阻气分	*shi zu qi fen*	dampness obstructing the qi division
湿阻中蕉	*shi zu zhong jiao*	dampness obstructing the middle burner
水不化气	*shui bu hua qi*	water not transforming the qi
痰火扰心	*tan huo rao xin*	phlegm fire harassing the heart
痰密心窍	*tan mi xin qiao*	phlegm confounding the portals of the heart
痰热阻肺	*tan re zu fei*	phlegm heat obstructs the lungs
痰湿阻肺	*tan shi zu fei*	phlegm dampness obstructing the lungs
痰阻肺络	*tan zu fei luo*	phlegm obstructing the lung network vessels
胃寒	*wei han*	stomach cold
胃火上升	*wei huo shang sheng*	stomach fire borne upward
卫气不固	*wei qi bu gu*	defensive qi not securing
胃气不和	*wei qi bu he*	stomach qi disharmony
胃气虚	*wei qi xu*	stomach qi vacuity
胃热	*wei re*	stomach heat
胃热壅盛	*wei re yong sheng*	stomach heat congesting & exuberant
胃失和降	*wei shi he jiang*	stomach loss of harmony & downbearing
胃虚	*wei xu*	stomach vacuity
胃阴虚	*wei yin xu*	stomach yin vacuity
温邪犯肺	*wen xie fan fei*	warm evils assailing the lungs
温邪上受	*wen xie shang shou*	warm evils affect above
下损及上	*xia sun ji shang*	lower detriment reaches above
相火妄动	*xiang huo wang dong*	ministerial fire frenetically stirring
小肠湿热	*xiao chang shi re*	small intestine damp heat

小肠虚寒	*xiao chang xu han*	small intestine vacuity cold
邪留三蕉	*xie liu san jiao*	evils retained in the three burners
心火亢盛	*xin huo kang sheng*	heart fire hyperactivity & exuberance
心火内炽	*xin huo nei chi*	heart fire blazing internally
心火上炎	*xin huo shang yan*	heart fire flares upward
心脾两虚	*xin pi liang xu*	heart-spleen dual vacuity
心气不宁	*xin qi bu ning*	heart qi not quiet
心气不缓	*xin qi bu shou*	heart qi not restraining
心肾不交	*xin shen bu jiao*	heart & kidneys not interacting
心虚胆怯	*xin xu dan qie*	heart vacuity, gallbladder timidity
心血虚	*xin xue xu*	heart blood vacuity
心阳虚	*xin yang xu*	heart yang vacuity
心阴虚	*xin yin xu*	heart yin vacuity
虚凤内动	*xu feng nei dong*	vacuity wind stirring internally
虚热上炎	*xu re shang yan*	vacuity heat flares upward
虚阳上浮	*xu yang shang fu*	vacuous yang floats upward
血不归经	*xue bu gui jing*	blood not returning to the channels
血分热毒	*xue fen re du*	blood division heat toxins
血分瘀热	*xue fen yu re*	blood division static heat
血随气陷	*xue sui qi xian*	blood follows qi fall
阳盛阴伤	*yang sheng yin shang*	yang exuberance damages yin
阴虚肺燥	*yin xu fei zao*	yin vacuity lung dryness
阴虚阳亢	*yin xu yang kang*	yin vacuity yang hyperactivity
阴虚阳旺	*yin xu yang wang*	yin vacuity yang effulgence
阴阳两虚	*yin yang liang xu*	yin & yang dual vacuity
荥卫不和	*ying wei bu he*	constructive & defensive disharmony
瘀热在里	*yu re zai li*	stasis & heat located in the interior
燥气伤肺	*zao qi shang fei*	dry qi damaging the lungs
中气不足	*zhong qi bu zu*	central qi insufficiency
中气下陷	*zhong qi xia xian*	central qi downward fall
中阳不振	*zhong yang bu zhen*	central yang devitalized
壮热食气	*zhuang re shi qi*	strong fire eats the qi

Confirming hunches

As you go on trying to translate, you will sometimes think you know something, like the Pinyin spelling of a character, but not be quite sure. In that case, instead of starting from scratch and looking the character up from the radical, you can go to the Index of Syllables which is just behind the Character Index in your Chinese-English dictionary. In other words, if you think the character is spelled *bao*, you can look up *bao* in this Syllable Index and see is the character is there. If it is, then you can look up the character alphabetically by its Pinyin spelling. If not, then you do have to start from scratch, identify the radical, count the strokes in the radical, find the radical's number, count the remaining strokes, find the character in the Character Index, etc.

If the character appears to be part of a Chinese medicinal's name or acupuncture point name and you think you know what the medicinal or the point name is but are not absolutely certain, then look up the medicinal or point name in the foregoing cheat sheets and then see if the characters match. If they do, you've saved yourself some time. If they don't, then you need to start from scratch.

16
Basic Chinese Medical Vocabulary

In the Council of Colleges of Acupuncture & Oriental Medicine (CCAOM) draft curriculum for a Doctor of Oriental Medicine (DOM) degree, learning to read modern medical Chinese with the aid of a dictionary is one of the requirements. Included is the memorization of a basic 500 word Chinese medical vocabulary.[1] Below is my list of approximately 500 important Chinese medical words. I have arranged this list by topics. See if you can memorize 10 new characters per day from this list. Each day, write out the new characters several times apiece. You can also make flash cards to quiz yourself on both the old and new vocabulary. By the time you get through with this list, you will have a very useful core Chinese medical vocabulary. Some of these characters appear more than once in the lists below since they have different meanings in different contexts. In a number of cases, I have also given compound terms where the medical meaning of a single character might not be otherwise self-evident.

Yin yang

阴	*yin*
阳	*yang*

Three powers (三才, *san cai*)

天	*tian*	heaven
人	*ren*	humanity
地	*di*	earth

Five phases (五行, *wu xing*)

木	*mu*	wood
火	*huo*	fire
土	*tu*	earth
金	*jin*	metal
水	*shui*	water
相	*xiang*	mutually
生	*sheng*	engendering
克	*ke*	restraining
母	*mu*	mother
子	*zi*	child
四时	*si shi*	four seasons, literally the four times
长夏	*chang xia*	long summer

---

[1] This has since been voted out of the DOM degree curriculum—a huge mistake!

Three treasures (三宝 , *san bao*) plus related terms

气	*qi*	
荣	*ying*	constructive
卫	*wei*	defensive
元气	*yuan qi*	source qi
宗气	*zong qi*	ancestral or chest qi
清气	*qing qi*	clear qi
浊气	*zuo qi*	turbid qi
谷气	*gu qi*	grain qi
中气	*zhong qi*	middle [burner] qi
血	*xue*	blood
精	*jing*	essence
神	*shen*	spirit
魂	*hun*	ethereal soul
魄	*po*	corporeal soul
津	*jin*	fluids
液	*ye*	humors
髓	*sui*	marrow
气海	*qi hai*	sea of qi
血海	*xue hai*	sea of blood
髓海	*sui hai*	sea of marrow, *i.e.*, the brain

Viscera & bowels (脏腑, *zang fu*) plus related terms

脏	*zang*	viscus/viscera
腑	*fu*	bowel/bowels
肝	*gan*	liver
心	*xin*	heart
脾	*pi*	spleen
肺	*fei*	lungs
肾	*shen*	kidneys
胆	*dan*	gallbladder
小肠	*xiao chang*	small intestine
胃	*wei*	stomach
大肠	*da chang*	large intestine
膀胱	*pang guang*	bladder
心包	*xin bao*	pericardium
三蕉	*san jiao*	triple burner
上蕉	*shang jiao*	upper burner
中蕉	*zhong jiao*	middle burner
下蕉	*xia jiao*	lower burner

脑	*nao*	brain
子宫	*zi gong*	uterus, literally the child palace
阴器	*yin qi*	genital organs
外阴	*wai yin*	external yin, *i.e.*, external genitalia
血室	*xue shi*	blood chamber
丹田	*dan tian*	field of cinnabar
相火	*xiang huo*	ministerial fire
君火	*jun huo*	sovereign fire
命门	*ming men*	life gate

Channels & vessels (经脉, *jing mai*)

经	*jing*	channel/channels
络	*luo*	network vessels
脉	*mai*	vessel/vessels
太阳	*tai yang*	greater yang
阳明	*yang ming*	yang brightness
少阳	*shao yang*	lesser yang
太阴	*tai yin*	greater yin
少阴	*shao yin*	lesser yin
厥阴	*jue yin*	end of yin
督脉	*du mai*	governing vessel
任脉	*ren mai*	conception vessel[2]
冲脉	*chong mai*	penetrating vessel
带脉	*dai mai*	girdling vessel
正经	*zheng jing*	regular channels
奇经	*qi jing*	extraordinary channels
八脉	*ba mai*	eight vessels
孙络	*sun luo*	grandchild network vessels
大络	*da luo*	great network vessel

Acupuncture points (穴位, *xue wei*)

穴	*xue*	point, literally a cave
井	*jing*	well
荥	*ying*	brook
输	*shu*	stream
经	*jing*	river
合	*he*	uniting

---

[2] Wiseman's new term for *ren mai* is the controlling vessel. Although this is an acceptable translation, I prefer to stick with the older conception vessel. The word *ren* can mean conception and this name is very entrenched. Since it is an acceptable translation, I see no reason to try to buck the tide on this one.

原	*yuan*	source
会	*hui*	meeting
交会	*jiao hui*	intersection
阿是穴	*a shi xue*	ouch point
募穴	*mu xue*	alarm point
输穴	*shu xue*	transport point
郄穴	*xi xue*	cleft point
夹脊	*jia ji*	paravertebral
十宣	*Shi Xuan*	10 Diffusers
八邪	*Ba Xie*	Eight Evils
八风	*Ba Feng*	Eight Winds

Eight principles (八纲, *ba gang*)

热	*re*	hot
寒	*han*	cold
表	*biao*	interior
里	*li*	exterior
虚	*xu*	vacuous/vacuity
实	*shi*	replete/repletion
阴	*yin*	
阳	*yang*	

Disease causes (病因, *bing yin*) plus related terms

内因	*nei yin*	internal causes
外因	*wai yin*	external causes
不内不外因	*bu nei bu wai yin*	neither internal nor external causes
内伤	*nei shang*	internal damage
外伤	*wai shang*	external damage
劳	*lao*	taxation
房劳	*fang lao*	bedroom, *i.e.,* sexual, taxation
正气	*zheng qi*	correct or righteous qi
邪气	*xie qi*	evil or pathogenic qi

Six environmmental excesses (六淫, *liu yin*) plus related terms

凤	*feng*	wind
湿	*shi*	dampness
燥	*zao*	dryness
署	*shu*	summerheat
热	*re*	heat
寒	*han*	cold

火	*huo*	fire
疠气	*li qi*	pestilential qi
疫气	*yi qi*	epidemic qi
时邪	*shi xie*	seasonal evils, literally time evils
虚邪	*xu xie*	vacuity evils
实邪	*shi xie*	replete evils
奇邪	*qi xie*	extraordinary evils
清邪	*qing xie*	clear evils
浊邪	*zuo xie*	turbid evils
客邪	*ke xie*	guest evils
合邪	*he xie*	combined evils
外感	*wai gan*	external affections or contractions
新感	*xin gan*	new affections
伏邪	*fu xie*	deep-lying or hidden evils
伤	*shang*	damage
毒	*du*	toxins
恶气	*e qi*	malign qi

Seven affects (七情, *qi qing*) plus related terms

怒	*nu*	anger
喜	*xi*	joy, excitment
思	*si*	thinking, thought
悲	*bei*	sorrow
惊	*jing*	fright
恐	*kong*	fear
哀	*ai*	grief
忧	*you*	anxiety

Tissues & anatomy

体	*ti*	body
形	*xing*	form
皮	*pi*	skin
毛	*mao*	hair
肌	*ji*	muscles
肉	*rou*	flesh
腠理	*cou li*	interstices
筋	*jin*	sinews
骨	*gu*	bones
目	*mu*	eyes
耳	*er*	ears
鼻	*bi*	nose

口	*kou*	mouth
齿	*chi*	teeth
舌	*she*	tongue
咽	*yan*	pharynx
喉	*hou*	larynx
咽喉	*yan hou*	throat
腹	*fu*	abdomen
大腹	*da fu*	large abdomen, *i.e.*, upper abdomen
腕	*wan*	venter
胃腕	*wei wan*	stomach venter
上腕	*shang wan*	upper venter
中腕	*zhong wan*	middle venter
下腕	*xia wan*	lower venter
少腹	*shao fu*	lesser abdomen, *i.e.*, lower abdomen
小腹	*xiao fu*	little abdomen, *i.e.*, lower abdomen
二阴	*er yin*	two yin, *i.e.*, the anus and urethra
前阴	*qian yin*	front yin, *i.e.*, urethra
后阴	*hou yin*	back yin, *i.e.*, anus
胁	*xie*	rib-side
腰	*yao*	lumbus
膝	*xi*	knees
背	*bei*	back
脊	*ji*	spine
手	*shou*	hand
足	*zu*	foot
肢	*zhi*	limb, extremity
脂	*zhi*	fat
乳	*ru*	breast

General concepts

先天	*xian tian*	former heaven, *i.e.*, prenatal
后天	*hou tian*	latter heaven, *i.e.*, postnatal
应	*ying*	correspondence
气化	*qi hua*	qi transformation
气机	*qi ji*	qi mechanism
病机	*bing ji*	disease mechanism
病里	*bing li*	pathology
运	*yun*	to move
化	*hua*	to transform
郁	*yu*	depression
滞	*zhi*	stagnation
瘀	*yu*	stasis

结	*jie*	binding
症	*zheng*	concretions
瘕	*jia*	conglomerations
积	*ji*	accumulations
聚	*ju*	gatherings
癖	*pi*	glomus
痰	*tan*	phlegm
饮	*yin*	rheum
虫	*chong*	insects, parasites
尿	*niao*	urine
小便	*xiao bian*	urination
大便	*da bian*	defecation
二便	*er bian*	the two excretions
逆	*ni*	counterflow
厥	*jue*	reversal
脱	*tuo*	desertion
陷	*xian*	fall
亡	*wang*	collapse
妄	*wang*	frenetic
盛	*sheng*	exuberance
旺	*wang*	effulgence
亏	*kui*	depletion
竭	*jie*	exhaustion
衰	*shuai*	debility
升	*sheng*	upbearing
降	*jiang*	downbearing
痹	*bi*	impediment
塞	*sai*	blockage
阻	*zu*	obstruction
壅	*yong*	congestion
凝	*ning*	congelation
停	*ting*	collect
崩	*beng*	flooding
漏	*lou*	leaking
月经	*yue jing*	menstruation, literally moon flow

Diseases (病, *bing*) & symptoms (症候, *zheng hou*)

疟	*nue*	malaria-like disease
疝	*shan*	mounting
肖渴	*xiao ke*	wasting thirst or wasting & thirsting
霍乱	*huo luan*	cholera-like disease
痒	*yang*	itching

疮	*chuang*	sores
痈	*yong*	welling absceses
疽	*ju*	flat abscesses
眩	*xuan*	vertigo
晕	*yun*	dizziness
肿	*zhong*	swelling
痛	*tong*	pain
疼	*teng*	aching
酸	*suan*	soreness
胀	*zhang*	distention
满	*man*	fullness
闷	*men*	oppression
癖	*pi*	glomus
沤吐	*ou tu*	vomiting
咳嗽	*ke sou*	coughing
哮	*xiao*	wheezing
喘	*chuan*	panting
汗	*han*	sweating
自汗	*zi han*	spontaneous sweating
盗汗	*dao han*	night sweats, literally thief sweating
感冒	*gan mao*	common cold or flu
潮热	*chao re*	tidal fever
烦	*fan*	vexation
躁	*zao*	agitation
泻痢	*xie li*	diarrhea & dysentery
泻泄	*xie xie*	diarrhea
便秘	*bian bi*	constipation
疸	*dan*	jaundice
疹	*zhen*	rash
狂	*kuang*	mania
癫	*dian*	withdrawal
渴	*ke*	thirst
痉	*jing*	tetany
痫	*xian*	epilepsy
痿	*wei*	wilting
反恶	*fan e*	nausea
恶逆	*e ni*	hiccup
淋	*lin*	strangury
疳	*gan*	gan
核	*he*	kernel or node
带下	*dai xia*	abnormal vaginal discharge
慢性	*man xing*	chronic
急性	*ji xing*	acute

Diagnosis (诊断 , *zhen duan*)

诊	*zhen*	examination
望	*wang*	inspection
苔	*tai*	fur
腻	*ni*	slimy
腐	*fu*	beancurd dregs-like
剥	*bo*	peeled
光	*guang*	bare
问	*wen*	inquiry
闻	*wen*	listening & smelling
腥	*xing*	fishy-smelling
臭	*chou*	malodorous
切	*qie*	palpation
寸	*cun*	inch
关	*guan*	bar
尺	*chi*	cubit
浮	*fu*	floating or superficial
沉	*chen*	sunken[3]
迟	*chi*	slow
数	*shu*	rapid
滑	*hua*	slippery when it has to do with the pulse, glossy when it has to do with the tongue fur
涩	*se*	choppy or rough
弦	*xian*	stringlike or bowstringlike
微	*wei*	faint
洪	*hong*	surging
紧	*jin*	tight
缓	*huan*	moderate or relaxed
芤	*kou*	scallion stalk-like
革	*ge*	drumskin-like
牢	*lao*	confined
濡	*ru*	soggy
软	*ruan*	soft
弱	*ruo*	weak
散	*san*	scattered or dissipated
细	*xi*	fine or thready
伏	*fu*	deep-lying or hidden
动	*dong*	stirring
促	*cu*	skipping
结	*jie*	bound

---

[3] Wiseman has recently changed this from deep to sunken in his *Practical Dictionary of Chinese Medicine*, Paradigm Publications, Brookline, MA 1998.

| 代 | *dai* | regularly irregular |
| 疾 | *ji* | racing |

Treatment methods (治法, *zhi fa*)

补	*bu*	supplement
泻	*xie*	drain
泄	*xie*	discharge
养	*yang*	nourish
滋	*zi*	enrich
除	*chu*	eliminate
去	*qu*	dispel
发	*fa*	emit
散	*san*	scatter or dissipate
肖	*xiao*	disperse
化	*hua*	transform
行	*xing*	move
霍	*huo*	quicken
理	*li*	rectify
调	*tiao*	regulate
平	*ping*	level or calm
安	*an*	quiet
宁	*ning*	quiet
镇	*zhen*	settle
熄	*xi*	extinguish
抑	*yi*	repress
潜	*qian*	subdue
止	*zhi*	stop or relieve
杀	*sha*	kill
下	*xia*	percipitate or descend
攻	*gong*	attack
扶	*fu*	support
润	*run*	moisten
生	*sheng*	engender
燥	*zao*	dry
通	*tong*	free the flow
利	*li*	disinhibit
渗	*shen*	percolate
宣	*xuan*	perfuse or diffuse
肃	*su*	depurate
托	*tuo*	out-thrust
固	*gu*	secure
涩	*se*	astringe

湿	*she*	contain
敛	*lian*	constrain
开	*kai*	open
宽	*kuan*	loosen
软	*ruan*	soften
和	*he*	harmonize
解	*jie*	resolve
清	*qing*	clear
壮	*zhuang*	strengthen
健	*jian*	fortify
益	*yi*	boost
助	*zhu*	assist or invigorate
凉	*liang*	cool
温	*wen*	warm
导	*dao*	abduct
培	*pei*	bank
疏	*shu*	course
舒	*shu*	soothe
柔	*rou*	emolliate
保	*bao*	protect
强	*qiang*	strengthen
破	*po*	break
涤	*di*	flush
救	*jiu*	stem or rescue
纳	*na*	grasp
引	*yin*	lead or guide
交	*jiao*	connect
催	*cui*	hasten
搜	*sou*	track

Formulas & medicinals (方药, *fang yao*)

方	*fang*	formula
药	*yao*	medicinal
草	*cao*	herb
剂	*ji*	Measure word for prescriptions or processed medicinals
复方	*fu fang*	compound prescription
单方	*dan fang*	simple prescription
煎	*jian*	decoction
饮	*yin*	drink or beverage
丸	*wan*	pill
散	*san*	powder
汤	*tang*	decoction or soup

膏	*gao*	ointment, paste, or plaster
丹	*dan*	elixir
茶	*cha*	tea
粥	*zhou*	porridge
酒	*jiu*	wine, alcohol
胶	*jiao*	gelatin
曲	*qu*	fermentation
片	*pian*	tablet
冲剂	*chong ji*	soluble granules
合剂	*he ji*	mixture
本草	*ben cao*	materia medica
味	*wei*	flavor
性	*xing*	nature
归经	*gui jing*	channel entry
服	*fu*	to administer, take, or dose
冲服	*chong fu*	administer after infusion
先煎	*xian jian*	decoct first
后下	*hou xia*	add after
包	*bao*	packet
炮	*pao*	blast-fry
炒	*chao*	stir-fry
煅	*duan*	calcine
蕉	*jiao*	scorch
煨	*wei*	roast
烘	*hong*	bake
炙	*zhi*	mix-fry
蒸	*zheng*	steam
煮	*zhu*	boil
熬	*ao*	simmer
灰	*hui*	ash
炭	*tan*	carbonize

Acupuncture & moxibustion (针灸, *zhen jiu*)

针	*zhen*	needle, acupuncture
灸	*jiu*	to burn, moxa, moxibustion
主穴	*zhu xue*	main or ruling points
火针	*huo zhen*	fire needle
温针	*wen zhen*	warm needle
皮肤针	*pi fu zhen*	dermal needle
电针	*dian zhen*	electroacupuncture
体针	*ti zhen*	body acupuncture
耳针	*er zhen*	ear acupuncture

耗针	*hao zhen*	fine needle
进针	*jin zhen*	inserting the needle
捻针	*nian zhen*	twirling the needle
留针	*liu zhen*	retaining the needle
手法	*shou fa*	hand technique
运针	*yun zhen*	moving or manipulating the needle
出针	*chu zhen*	removing the needle
经刺	*jing ci*	channel puncture
络刺	*luo ci*	network vessel puncture
晕针	*yun zhen*	dizziness or fainting during needling
折针	*zhe zhen*	broken needle
滞针	*zhi zhen*	stuck needle, literally stagnant needle
得气	*de qi*	to obtain the qi
导气	*dao qi*	to abduct or lead the qi
艾炷灸	*ai zhu jiu*	mugwort moxa with cones
艾条灸	*ai tiao jiu*	mugwort moxa with a roll
灯心灸	*deng xin jiu*	juncus moxa
拔罐法	*ba guan fa*	cupping

17
General Vocabulary

Only part of the words in a modern Chinese medical text or journal article are going to be technical medical terms. A number of the words are going to be non-technical words. While the focus of this workbook is specifically on translating modern medical Chinese, learning or at least becoming familiar with a number of non-technical terms can help make translation easier. Below are some words which you will see time and time again. If you memorize these, it will make your life as a translator easier in the long run. As with the technical medical vocabulary in the preceding chapter, these words are arranged according to topic.

Counting & numbers

Chinese use both Arabic numerals and their own way of writing numbers. Because of the scientific nature of the modern Chinese medical literature, numbers appear all the time in the form of data. They are also used when arranging a piece in outline form. Therefore, it is important to know how to read Chinese numbers.

一	*yi*	one
二	*er*	two
三	*san*	three
四	*si*	four
五	*wu*	five
六	*liu*	six
七	*qi*	seven
八	*ba*	eight
九	*jiu*	nine
十	*shi*	ten

Numbers 11-19 are made by adding 1-9 to 10.

十一	*shi yi*	11
十二	*shi er*	12
十三	*shi san*	13
十四	*shi si*	14
十五	*shi wu*	15
十六	*shi liu*	16
十七	*shi qi*	17
十八	*shi ba*	18
十九	*shi jiu*	19

Twenty is made by writing 2 [x] 10, *i.e.*, 二十 (*er shi*, 20). Therefore, 21-29 are written:

二十一	*er shi yi*	21
二十二	*er shi er*	22
二十三	*er shi san*	23
二十四	*er shi si*	24
二十五	*er shi wu*	25
二十六	*er shi liu*	26
二十七	*er shi qi*	27
二十八	*er shi ba*	28
二十九	*er shi jiu*	29

Numbers 30-90 are written in the corresponding way:

三十	*san shi*	30
三十一	*san shi yi*	31
三十二	*san shi er*	32
四十	*si shi*	40
四十一	*si shi yi*	41
五十	*wu shi*	50
六十	*liu shi*	60
七十	*qi shi*	70
八十	*ba shi*	80
九十	*jiu shi*	90

The number 100 is written 百 (*bai*). Therefore, 二百三十 (*er bai san shi*) equals 230. 三百五十八 (*san bai wu shi ba*) equals 358.

The number 1,000 is written 千 (*qian*). Therefore, 四千五百五十六 (*si qian wu bai wu shi liu*) equals 4,556. 三千九百 (*san qian jiu bai*) equals 3,900. 二千二 (*er qian er*) equals 2,002.

The number 10,000 is written 万 (*wan*). Therefore, 二万 (*er wan*) equals 20,000. 三万一千二百八十八 (*san wan yi qian er bai ba shi ba*) equals 31, 288.

Exercise. Please write the Arabic numerals for each of these Chinese numbers. Cover the answers first and then check the answers after you have completed the exercise.

A. 九十   (*jiu shi*)
B. 一百一   (*yi bai yi*)
C. 三千二百三十八   (*san qian er bai san shi ba*)
D. 二万三千一百一   (*er wan san qian yi bai yi*)
E. 一千七百五十三   (*yi qian qi bai wu shi san*)
F. 三十六   (*san shi liu*)
G. 九十九   (*jiu shi jiu*)
H. 七百二十二   (*qi bai er shi er*)
I. 十五   (*shi wu*)

J. 五十   (*wu shi*)

Answers: A. 90; B. 101; C. 3,238; D. 23,101; E. 1,853; F. 36; G. 99; H. 722; I. 15; J. 50

Further:

One million is 一百万 (*yi bai wan*).
Ten million is 一千万 (*yi qian wan*).
One hundred million is 一万万 (*yi wan wan*).
And one billion is 十万万 (*shi wan wan*).

All the above numbers are cardinals. When it comes to ordinals, *i.e.*, first, second, third, fifty-first, etc. the character 弟(*di*) is simply put in front of the number. Therefore:

弟一	*di yi*	first
弟二	*di er*	second
弟三	*di san*	third
弟四	*di si*	fourth
弟五	*di wu*	fifth
弟六	*di liu*	sixth
弟十一	*di shi yi*	11th
弟百一	*di bai yi*	101st
弟千五百九十一	*di qian wu bai jiu shi yi*	1,591st

Dates

It is not uncommon in case histories and clinical reports to come across dates. The word 年 (*nian*) means year. The word 月(*yue*, moon) also means month, while the word 日(*ri*, sun) also means day. Therefore, can you figure out the following date: 1975 年 7 月 5 日? The answer is July 5, 1975. Below is the way Chinese write the 12 months of the year:

一月	*yi yue*	January
二月	*er yue*	February
三月	*san yue*	March
四月	*si yue*	April
五月	*wu yue*	May
六月	*liu yue*	June
七月	*qi yue*	July
八月	*ba yue*	August
九月	*jiu yue*	September
十月	*shi yue*	October
十一月	*shi yi yue*	November
十二月	*shi er yue*	December

Exercise. Try reading the following dates. Cover the answers until you are through and then check them against your own.

A. 1946 年　2 月　20 日
B. 1956 年　8 月　1 日
C. 1997 年　9 月　29 日
D. 1964 年　10 月　6 日
E. 1985 年　1 月　15 日

Answers: A. Feb. 20, 1946; B. Aug. 1, 1956; C. Sept. 29, 1997; D. Oct. 6, 1964; E. Jan. 15, 1985

The days of the week are written as follows:

星期天	*xing qi tian*	Sunday
星期一	*xing qi yi*	Monday
星期二	*xing qi er*	Tuesday
星期三	*xing qi san*	Wednesday
星期四	*xing qi si*	Thursday
星期五	*xing qi wu*	Friday
星期六	*xing qi liu*	Saturday

Sometimes, Sunday is also written 星期日 (*xing qi ri*), literally sun day.

Time

钟	(*zhong*) means time as told by a clock.
分钟	(*fen zhong*) means minutes.
六点钟	(*liu dian zhong*) means six o'clock.
十分钟	(*shi fen zhong*) means 10 minutes.
小时	(*xiao shi*) means hour.
上午	(*shang wu*) means AM.
下午	(*xia wu*) means PM.
今	(*jin*) means recent, not, presently.
古	(*gu*) means ancient.
今代	(*jin dai*) means modern.
古人	(*gu ren*) means ancient people, the ancients.

Positions in space

上	*shang*	up
下	*xia*	down
中	*zhong*	middle
左	*zuo*	left
右	*you*	right

东	*dong*	east
西	*xi*	west
南	*nan*	south
北	*bei*	north
东北	*dong bei*	northeast, but literally east north
西北	*xi bei*	northwest, but literally west north
西南	*xi nan*	southwest, but literally west south
东南	*dong nan*	southeast, but literally east south
里	*li*	inside
外	*wai*	outside
前	*qian*	in front of, before
后	*hou*	behind, in back of
在	*zai*	to be located at
到	*dao*	to reach, to arrive at
住	*zhu*	to reside, to stay

Place names

中国	*Zhong Guo*	China, literally Middle Country
美国	*Mei Guo*	U.S.A., literally Beautiful Country
四川	*Si Chuan*	literally Four Rivers
云南	*Yun Nan*	literally Clouds South
山东	*Shan Dong*	literally Moutain East
山西	*Shan Xi*	literally Moutain West
西安	*Xi An*	literally Western Peace
上海	*Shang Hai*	literally Above the Sea
海南	*Hai Nan*	literally Sea South
东海	*Dong Hai*	literally Eastern Sea
北海	*Bei Hai*	literally Northern Sea
北京	*Bei Jing*	literally Northern Capital
南京	*Nan Jing*	literally Southern Capital
广东	*Guang Dong*	literally Vast East
广西	*Guang Xi*	literally Vast West
广州	*Guang Zhou*	
杭州	*Huang Zhou*	
苏州	*Su Zhou*	
福州	*Fu Zhou*	

The last four names on this list are all names of cities in China. The character 州(*zhou*) is translated as river island by Wiseman. Remember that 四川 (*si chuan*) literally means four rivers. So the character 川 (*chuan*) means river. In the case of *zhou*, we have the character for river with three dots in-between the lines of the picture of a flowing river. These three dots are as if islands in the middle of a river, and many early Chinese cities were built for defensive reasons on such rivers. However, nowadays, this ending simply denotes the name of city or geographic region.

In the People's Republic of China, there is the tendency to run place names together, so that *Bei Jing* becomes Beijing, *Si Chuan* becomes Sichuan, and *Guang Dong* becomes Guangdong. Chinese say that these compound terms are really a single "word." This argument underscores the fundamental differences between Chinese and English. A single concept or entity is not necessarily a single word in English. For instance, we do not write Newjersey, Newyork, Northdakota, or Cedarrapids. Therefore, as a native English speaker, I believe the Chinese are wrong when they write place names in Pinyin by running the character pronunciations all together, as in Shanghai, Nanjing, and Yunnan.

Historical periods

夏	*Xia*	2205-1766 BCE
商	*Shang*	1766-1122 BCE
周	*Zhou*	1122-770 BCE
春秋	*Chun Qiu* (Spring & Autumn)	770-476 BCE
战国	*Zhan Guo* (Warring States)	476-221 BCE
秦	*Qin*	221-206 BCE
汉	*Han*	206 BCE - 220 CE
三国	*San Guo* (Three Kingdoms)	220-265 CE
西晋	*Xi Jin* (Western Jin)	265-316 CE
东晋	*Dong Jin* (Eastern Jin)	317-420 CE
南北朝	*Nan Bei Chao* (Southern & Northern Period)	420-589 CE
隋	*Sui*	589-618 CE
唐	*Tang*	618-907 CE
五代	*Wu Dai* (Five Dynasties)	907-960 CE
北宋	*Bei Song* (Northern Song)	960-1127 CE
南宋	*Nan Song* (Southern Song)	1127-1279 CE
辽	*Liao*	916-1125 CE
叫	*Jin*	1115-1234 CE
元	*Yuan*	1280-1368 CE
明	*Ming*	1368-1644 CE
清	*Qing*	1644-1911 CE
中华民国	*Zhong Hua Min Guo* (Republic of China)	1912-1949 (on the mainland)
中华人民共和国	*Zhong Hua Ren Min Gong He Guo* (People's Republic of China) 1949-	
代	*dai,* dynasty	

People's names

Chinese have two basic kinds of names: 名 (*ming*) and 字 (*zi*). A person's *ming* is their name at birth. This name is comprised of two parts. There is the family name, what we call our surname, and there is the given or personal name. In English we talk about our first and last names. Our first name is our given or personal name, while our last name is our family name or surname. In China, it is just the other way around. A person's family name comes first, followed by their personal name. There are approximately 100 different Chinese family names in common use. Only a bare handful of these have two syllables. The overwhelming majority of family names have only a single syllable. Personal names tend to be compound terms made up of two characters. These two characters, *or words*, are picked, at least in part for the meaning they convey. Therefore, Chinese personal names are very much like typical American Indian names, they mean something which hopefully the person will grow to embody. A minority of Chinese only have a single personal name.

Usually, authors' names on books and journal articles are easy to identify. They are typically set off typographically in some way. However, when a Chinese person's name is embedded in text, the beginning translator may look up all three characters and not know that they are dealing with a person's name. Yet the meaning of the three characters means absolutely nothing in the context the translation. What to do?

Please look up the character 革 (*ge*) in your Chinese-English dictionary. Under its definitions, you will see 1) leather, hide; 2) change, transformation; 3) remove from office, expel; and 4) a surname. If you come across a two or three character combination which means absolutely nothing comprehensible, check and see if the first character can be a surname. If so, then see if the other one or two characters make sense as the rest of the name. For instance, the words 曰 (*yue*) and 云 (*yun*) both means "to say". If these are followed by a colon or words in quotation marks of some kind, it is possible the characters in front of either of these two words you are having such trouble with are actually someone's name. For instance, 丹溪曰: means, "Dan-xi said:..."

Other times you may see a single character followed by the word 师, teacher. Thus 王师 means "Teacher Wang". 氏 means "master or mister". Hence 陈氏 means "Master or Mister Chen". 老医 means "old doctor", while 老中医 means "old Chinese doctor". Sometimes one will see either of these two titles of respect after a single family name first, such as 孙老医, "Old Doctor Sun". If one is not an Old Doctor, they might be referred to as simply 高医 or 高医生, both of which mean "Dr. Gao".

As you become more practiced at translating Chinese, you will come to recognize some of the most commonly occurring Chinese family names. Below is a list of frequently seen family names:

安	An		卞	Bian		晁	Chao
敖	Ao		并	Bing		车	Che
巴	Ba		卜	Bu		陈	Chen
包	Bao		蔡	Cai		程	Cheng
贝	Bei		曹	Cao		池	Chi
边	Bian		常	Chang		春	Chun

崔	Cui	郦	Li	山	Shan		
戴	Dai	连	Lian	商	Shang		
党	Dang	林	Lin	邵	Shao		
邓	Deng	柳	Liu	申	Shen		
丁	Ding	卢	Lu	沈	Shen		
董	Dong	陆	Lu	盛	Sheng		
杜	Du	路	Lu	师	Shi		
段	Duan	马	Ma	寿	Shou		
范	Fan	满	Man	帅	Shuai		
方	Fang	毛	Mao	水	Shui		
费	Fei	孟	Meng	司	Si		
丰	Feng	米	Mi	松	Song		
冯	Feng	苗	Miao	宋	Song		
符	Fu	缪	Miao	苏	Su		
盖	Gai	闵	Min	隋	Sui		
甘	Gan	明	Ming	索	Suo		
高	Gao	莫	Mo	邰	Tai		
戈	Ge	墨	Mo	覃	Tan		
革	Ge	穆	Mu	唐	Tang		
公	Gong	聂	Nie	汤	Tang		
古	Gu	区	Ou	陶	Tao		
关	Guan	潘	Pan	滕	Teng		
贯	Guan	盘	Pan	田	Tian		
归	Gui	庞	Pang	铁	Tie		
过	Guo	彭	Peng	佟	Tong		
国	Guo	皮	Pi	童	Tong		
海	Hai	平	Ping	汪	Wang		
何	He	朴	Po	王	Wang		
贺	He	戚	Qi	翁	Weng		
赫	He	齐	Qi	乌	Wu		
洪	Hong	祁	Qi	邬	Wu		
华	Hua	乔	Qiao	习	Xi		
黄	Huang	秦	Qin	席	Xi		
计	Ji	庆	Qing	相	Xiang		
江	Jiang	邱	Qiu	向	Xiang		
金	Jin	仇	Qiu	肖	Xiao		
康	Kang	曲	Qu	谢	Xie		
科	Ke	权	Quan	辛	Xin		
匡	Kuang	全	Quan	邢	Xing		
邝	Kuang	冉	Ran	薛	Xue		
赖	Lai	饶	Rao	荀	Xun		
劳	Lao	戎	Rong	严	Yan		
老	Lao	荣	Rong	羊	Yang		

杨	Yang	元	Yuan	朱	Zhu		
叶	Ye	原	Yuan	竺	Zhu		
易	Yi	乐	Yue	祝	Zhu		
殷	Yin	云	Yun	庄	Zhuang		
尹	Yin	曾	Zeng	卓	Zhuo		
印	Yin	展	Zhan	宗	Zong		
应	Ying	张	Zhang	邹	Zou		
英	Ying	赵	Zhao	祖	Zu		
游	You	甄	Zhen	左	Zuo		
余	Yu	郑	Zheng				
虞	Yu	支	Zhi				
郁	Yu	钟	Zhong				
喻	Yu	周	Zhou				

A person's *zi* name (字) is their so-called style name. This is a name which is taken at 20 years of age. It is something similar to a *nom de plume* or pen-name. In fact, some Chinese have different *zi* names as they go through life, each *zi* name saying something about that person at that stage of life. For instance, two of the four great masters of medicine of the Jin-yuan dynasties were Li Gao and Zhu Zhen-heng. These were their given names. Later on, Li became known as Dong Yuan, while Zhu was given or took the *zi* name Dan Xi, Cinnabar Creek. Typically, *zi* names are made up of two characters.

Sometimes you will come across an author's name one or more characters of which you cannot find in your Chinese-English dictionary. This is because given names are given because of their meaning, their sound, and even the auspicious number of strokes in their characters. So some Chinese have names made up from very archaic or abstruse characters. When you come across a name character which you cannot find in your simplified, Pinyin Chinese-English dictionary from the PRC, my suggestion is that you look the word up in *Mathew's Chinese English Dictionary*. As you hopefully will remember, *Mathew's* is the most commonly used complicated or old character Chinese-English dictionary. This dictionary is much more complete when it comes to the number of characters it contains than the typical Pinyin Chinese-English dictionary, and you can usually find name characters in this dictionary which you cannot in your simplified dictionary. I will discuss how to look characters up in *Matthew's* in a separate chapter below.

Just as I do not think we should run on place names like Beijing and Shanghai where the two characters actually each mean something, I also do not think we should run on Chinese personal names when writing them in English. In the PRC, the style of writing one's name in Pinyin is to write the family name first and then the two given names secondly run on into each other. Therefore, one gets Zhou Enlai, Mao Zedong, Zhang Zemin, etc. I prefer the method used in Taiwan and Hong Kong where the two given names are separated by a hyphen. This clearly alerts you to the fact of which is the family name and which is the given name, without running both together. My name in English is Robert Sutton Flaws. It is not Robertsutton Flaws. My wife's name in English is Honora Lee Wolfe, not Honoralee Wolfe. Similarly, I prefer Ma Ze-dong, Zhou En-lai, and Zhang Ze-min.

To make matters more complicated, Chinese like to invert their names when they come to the U.S. so that there is not so much confusion about which is the their family name. Therefore, were Mao Ze-dong to move to Boulder, CO today, it is likely he would write his name Zedong Mao or Ze Dong Mao. If you do not either run the two characters of the personal name together or separate them by a hyphen, things get very confusing when Chinese move to Western countries. Is Zhou En Lai Mr. Zhou or Mr. Lai?

Colors

白	*bai*	white
黑	*hei*	black
赤	*chi*	red
红	*hong*	red
绛	*jiang*	crimson
褐	*he*	brown
黄	*huang*	yellow
青	*qing*	blue or blue-green
紫	*zi*	purple
灰	*hui*	grey, ashen
绿	*lu*	green
色	*se*	color

Exercise: If 茶 (*cha*) is tea, 绿茶 (*lu cha*) is ______ tea and 红茶 (*hong cha*) is ______ tea. (Actually, this is what we would call black tea.) If 酒(*jiu*) means alcohol, then what kind of alcohol is 白酒 (*bai jiu*)? What kind is 黄酒 (*huang jiu*)?

Answers: Green tea; red tea; white alcohol (such as vodka and schnaaps), yellow alcohol (such as yellow rice wine or sake)

Common adjectives

好	*hao*	good
不好	*bu hao*	no good
很好	*hen hao*	very good
不太好	*bu tai hao*	not very good
不良	*bu liang*	not good
大	*da*	big
小	*xiao*	small
少	*shao*	scanty
多	*duo*	profuse, many
过	*guo*	super-, over-, excessive
过多	*guo duo*	excessive
高	*gao*	tall
短	*duan*	short, brief, lacking

长	*chang*	long
老	*lao*	old
青年	*qing nian*	young, literally green in years
难	*nan*	hard, difficult
易	*yi*	easy

Common things found in the Chinese medical literature

山	*shan*	mountain
日	*ri*	sun
月	*yue*	moon
海	*hai*	sea
江	*jiang*	river
林	*lin*	forest
石	*shi*	stone
电	*dian*	electricity
玉	*yu*	jade
田	*tian*	field
门	*men*	door
鱼	*yu*	fish
牛	*niu*	cow, ox
马	*ma*	horse
龙	*long*	dragon
凤	*feng*	phoenix
鸡	*ji*	chicken
狗	*gou*	dog
龟	*gui*	turtle
蛇	*she*	snake
虫	*chong*	worm, insect, parasite

Weights & measures

分	*fen*	tenth of an inch or tenth of a *qian*; see below
寸	*cun*	inch
尺	*chi*	foot or cubit
里	*li*	approx. 1km
厘米	*li mi*	centimeter
米	*mi*	meter
毫米	*hao mi*	millimeter
升	*sheng*	liter
毫升	*hao sheng*	milliliter
克	*ke*	gram
毫克	*hao ke*	milligram

公斤	*gong jin*	kilogram
钱	*qian*	approx. 3 grams
两	*liang*	10 *qian*
斤	*jin*	10 *liang*

Grammatical, function, or linking words

When it comes to looking up the meaning of Chinese medical technical terms, I recommend Nigel Wiseman's *English-Chinese Chinese-English Dictionary of Chinese Medicine*. However, when it comes to everyday, non-medical terms which are basically grammar words, sometimes looking these up in your regular Chinese-English dictionary may not be very helpful. Instead of defining these words in English, the dictionary may give a Chinese example of how the word is used. Without looking up every word in the example, this can be very frustrating.

The following is a list of commonly used grammatical, function, or linking words. Although this list is, by no means, exhaustive, hopefully it can help you shorten your work, especially as a beginner. Also included on this list are a number of non-medical abstract concepts which are frequently met in the Chinese medical literature. If you just look over this list and think about the meanings of the compound terms on it, you would learn a lot about the logic of the Chinese language. If you were to systematically memorize all the words in this list plus your specifically medical vocabulary given above, you would be able to read a huge amount of the Chinese medical literature with good comprehension.

挨次	*ai ci*	one after another, in turn
谙	*an*	be familiar with something
按	*an*	in accordance with
按期	*an qi*	on schedule
按时	*an shi*	on time
按照	*an zhao*	in accordance with
般	*ban*	kind, type
伴有	*ban you*	accompanied by
办法	*ban fa*	measure, method
帮助	*bang zhu*	assist
包含	*bao han*	include
包括	*bao kuo*	include
包括...在内	*bao kuo...zai nei*	include
保持	*bao chi*	maintain
保全	*bao quan*	preserve
保证	*bao zheng*	guarantee
倍	*bei*	double, multiply
倍加	*bei jia*	extra, more than usual
备用	*bei yong*	be used
本来	*ben lai*	originally

本身	*ben shen*	itself
本质	*ben zhi*	basic nature
比	*bi*	in comparison to
比较	*bi jiao*	relatively, comparatively
比如	*bi ru*	for example
毕竟	*bi jing*	finally, in the final analysis, when all is said and done
必	*bi*	must, inevitably
必	*bi ran*	definitely
必须	*bi xu*	must
必要	*bi yao*	necessary, essential
必由	*bi you*	essential, necessary
避	*bi*	avoid
便	*bian*	a particle indicating that the fact referred to next results from the fact immediately preceding
便是	*bian shi*	final particle emphasizing the preceding statement
变	*bian*	change
变端	*bian duan*	change
变	*bian hua*	change
变为	*bian wei*	change to
辨别	*bian bie*	distinguish
辨认	*bian ren*	distinguish
遍	*bian*	everywhere
标志	*biao zhi*	characteristic
表面上	*biao man shang*	on the surface, outside
表示	*biao shi*	indicate
表现	*biao xian*	manifest as
别	*bie*	additional, distinguish¬
别出	*bie chu*	offshoots
并	*bing*	simultaneous
并且	*bing qie*	and, moreover, furthermore
并提	*bing ti*	refer together
并用	*bing yong*	apply simultaneously
不	*bu*	not, no
不必	*bu bi*	not necessary, unnecessary
不单	*bu dan*	not only
不单…而	*bu dan…er…*	not only…but
不等	*bu deng*	not identical
不定	*bu ding*	unstable, uncertain
不断	*bu duan*	unceasingly, continuously
不光	*bu guang*	not only
不过	*bu guo*	however
不仅	*bu jin*	not only
不仅…并	*bu jin…bing…*	not only…also

不可	*bu ke*	not ok, cannot
不利于	*bu li yu*	not conducive to
不免	*bu mian*	inevitably
不全面	*bu quan mian*	incomplete
不时	*bu shi*	frequently, time and again
不同	*bu tong*	not the same, different
不问	*bu wen*	regardless whether
不一	*bu yi*	not one, different
不一定	*bu yi ding*	not necessarily
不宜	*bu yi*	should not
不予	*bu yu*	not to grant
不再	*bu zai*	not again, not any longer
不止	*bu zhi*	incessantly, without stop
部分	*bu fen*	element
部位	*bu wei*	location
才	*cai*	then, particle used to stress time
采取	*cai qu*	select
采用	*cai yong*	select
叁考	*can kao*	consult
侧	*ce*	side
曾	*ceng*	once, before, indicates a past occurrence
差不多	*cha bu duo*	almost, nearly
产生	*chan sheng*	produce
产物	*chan wu*	product
场所	*chang suo*	location
常	*chang*	often, regularly, commonly
常常	*chang chang*	often, regularly
常见	*chang jian*	commonly seen, often
常数	*chang shu*	constantly, regularly
常用	*chang yong*	regularly used, commonly used
长期	*chang qi*	long-term
长时期	*chang shi qi*	long-term
彻底	*che di*	carefully
称	*cheng*	designate, call
称号	*cheng hao*	title, designation
称为	*cheng wei*	call
称作	*cheng zuo*	be called, call
成	*cheng*	constitute
成倍	*cheng bei*	several times, several-fold
成年	*cheng nian*	year after year
成天	*cheng tian*	all day long, all the time
成为	*cheng wei*	constitute

呈	*cheng*	manifest, present
呈现	*cheng xian*	bring forth
乘	*cheng*	seize, exploit, take advantage of
程度	*cheng du*	degree
程序	*cheng xu*	sequence
承受	*cheng shou*	take, receive
重	*chong*	doubled
重复	*chong fu*	repeat, repetitive
初	*chu*	just before, initial
初步	*chu bu*	preliminary, literally, first step
初期	*chu qi*	initial phase
初起	*chu qi*	begin
出	*chu*	exit, leave
出发	*chu fa*	go out from, proceed from
出来	*chu lai*	come out, a particle indicating the outcome of a process indicated by the immediately preceding verb
出入	*chu ru*	difference
出现	*chu xian*	let appear, bring forth
出于	*chu yu*	leave from
除...外	*chu...wai...*	except for
除此以外	*chu ci yi wai*	in addition
除了	*chu le*	except for
除去不用	*chu qu bu yong*	omit altogether
处理	*chu li*	deal with, sort out, handle
处	*chu*	locality
传	*chuan*	transmit
传变	*chuan bian*	transmission & transformation
此	*ci*	this
此后	*ci hou*	henceforth, after this
此时	*ci shi*	at this time
此外	*ci wai*	furthermore
次	*ci*	-times
次序	*ci xu*	sequence
次要	*ci yao*	of secondary importance
次于	*ci yu*	be secondary to
从	*cong*	from
从...内	*cong... nei*	from within
从...入手	*cong...ru shou*	start from...
从...上	*cong... shang*	starting from..., on the basis of...
从...中	*cong...zhong*	from
从...来说	*cong...lai shuo*	as for ...
从此	*cong ci*	from this time onward, from now on
从而	*cong er*	hence, therefore

从来	*cong lai*	always, at all times
从属	*cong shu*	categorize
从头	*cong tou*	from the beginning
促使	*cu shi*	lead to
猝	*cu ran*	sudden
存在	*cun zai*	be present, exist
措	*cuo*	make use of
措施	*cuo shi*	measure, approach
措杂	*cuo za*	mixed
措综	*cuo zong*	complicated
措综复杂	*cuo zong fu za*	complex
达到	*da dao*	attain, reach
大抵	*da di*	for the most part, mostly
大都	*da du*	for the most part, mostly
大凡	*da fan*	in most cases, generally
大概	*da gai*	as a rule, most likely
大家	*da jia*	all, everybody
大体	*da ti*	on the whole, in the main, for the most part
大体上	*da ti shang*	in general
大约	*da yue*	in general, about, approximately
带	*dai*	carry along
带来	*dai lai*	cause, lead to
代表	*dai biao*	represent
代名词	*dai ming ci*	synonym
待	*dai*	wait
待到...以后	*dai dao...yi hou...*	after...
单	*dan*	only, solely
但	*dan*	but
但是	*dan shi*	however
当	*dang*	should, must
当...时	*dang... shi*	at the time when...
当	*dang ran*	of course
到	*dao*	to, with
到处	*dao chu*	everywhere, in all places
到达	*dao da*	reach
到底	*dao di*	in the end
道理	*dao li*	principle
得	*de*	receive, obtain
得出	*de chu*	get
的	*de*	possessive particle
等	*deng*	particle defining the end of a list
...等	*...deng*	etc.

等等	*deng deng*	and so on and so forth
等量	*deng liang*	equal amount
等于	*deng yu*	be comparable to
抵触	*di chu*	be in conflict
地步	*di bu*	condition, stage
地方	*di fang*	location, place
地	*di wei*	position
弟	*di*	particle indicating the following number is an ordinal
顶	*ding*	very, most, extremely
顶多	*ding duo*	at the most, at best
定出	*ding chu*	decide
定名	*ding ming*	name
定义	*ding yi*	define
懂得	*dong de*	understand
动态	*dong tai*	nature of movement
动作	*dong zuo*	movement
都	*dou*	all
都是	*dou shi*	always, all, in each case
独	*du*	alone, only
度	*du*	degree
端	*duan*	end point
对	*dui*	on, at
对比	*dui bi*	balance, comparison
对称	*dui chen*	symmetrical
对立	*dui li*	antagonistic
对于	*dui yu*	on
多	*duo*	many, often
多方	*duo fang*	in every way, spare no effort in doing something
多少	*duo shao*	amount
多数	*duo shu*	mostly, often
恶化	*e hua*	aggravate, aggravation
而	*er*	and
而后	*er hou*	then, afterwards
而且	*er qie*	moreover, in addition, but also
而已	*er yi*	and thereby ending
发	*fa*	develop, appear
发生	*fa sheng*	develop, generate
发现	*fa xian*	find, discover
发育	*fa yu*	development
发展	*fa zhan*	development
法度	*fa du*	law

法则	*fa ze*	rule
番	*fan*	measure word for activities
凡	*fan*	all
凡是	*fan shi*	all, every, without exception, whenever
反	*fan*	opposite
反常	*fan chang*	unusual
反复	*fan fu*	return, repeat
反过来	*fan guo lai*	conversely
反来	*fan lai*	conversely, on the contrary
反映	*fan ying*	appear, be reflected in
反应	*fan ying*	reaction
反之	*fan zhi*	in contrast
范畴	*fan chou*	realm, category
范围	*fan wei*	spectrum
方才	*fang cai*	then
方面	*fang mian*	aspect
...方面	*...fang mian*	as for...
方向	*fang xiang*	orientation
方针	*fang zhen*	approach
防	*fang*	prevent
防止	*fang zhi*	prevent
放	*fang*	let
非	*fei*	be not
非...不可	*fei...bu ke*	impossible if not...
非...不...	*fei...bu...*	only if...is...
非但...而且	*fei dan... er qie*	not only...but also
分	*fen*	differentiate, divide
分辨	*fen bian*	differentiate
分别	*fen bie*	differentiate, respectively, separately
分不出	*fen bu chu*	impossible to distinguish
分部	*fen bu*	individual regions
分开	*fen kai*	separately
分类	*fen lei*	categorize
分离	*fen li*	separate
分配	*fen pei*	associate separately with
分属	*fen shu*	assign
分为	*fen wei*	divide into
分析	*fen xi*	analyze
分有	*fen you*	distinguish
分作	*fen zuo*	categorize
否	*fou*	no, not
否认	*fou ren*	deny
否则	*fou ze*	if not then, otherwise

副作用	*fu zuo yong*	side effect
复	*fu*	return
复来	*fu lai*	return
复杂	*fu za*	complicated, complex
改	*gai*	change
改变	*gai bian*	change
改善	*gai shan*	improve
改为	*gai wei*	replace by
概	*gai*	in general, in sum
概况	*gai kuang*	rough survey
概括	*gai kuo*	outline
概括性	*gai kuo xing*	general
感	*gan*	to be affected
感受	*gan shou*	to be affected by
纲领	*gang ling*	guiding principle
纲要	*gang yao*	fundamental categories
高低	*gao di*	level
各	*ge*	indicates that each individual of a group does/is the same thing
个人	*ge ren*	each person
各个	*ge ge*	each
个	*ge*	a general measure word
根据	*gen ju*	on the basis of
根源	*gen yuan*	basic source
跟着	*gen zhe*	following, and immediately afterwards
更	*geng*	more, even more, further
更...一步	*geng...yi bu*	even more...
更好	*geng hao*	better
工作	*gong zuo*	work, activity
功夫	*gong fu*	effort, work
功能	*gong neng*	function
功效	*gong xiao*	efficacy
共	*gong*	altogether, in all, in total
构成	*gou cheng*	constitute
孤立	*gu li*	isolate
古	*gu*	ancient
古人	*gu ren*	ancient person
古为今用	*gu wei jin yong*	make the old useful for today
故	*gu*	hence, therefore, so
顾	*gu*	observe
固定	*gu ding*	identify definitely
怪	*guai*	uncommon, very, quite, rather
关	*guan*	affect, concern

关键	*guan jian*	key point
关键性	*guan jian xing*	central, essential
关系	*guan xi*	relationship
关于	*guan yu*	as regards
观察	*guan cha*	observe
贯串	*guan chuan*	permeate, penetrate
广泛	*guang fan*	extensive, comprehensive
广义	*guang yi*	broad sense
归	*gui*	identify as
归类	*gui lei*	categorize
归纳	*gui na*	draw inductive conclusions
归入	*gui ru*	associate with
归属	*gui shu*	belong to
归于	*gui yu*	turn to, associate with
过	*guo*	excessive, too much, undue
过程	*guo cheng*	process
过度	*guo du*	excessive
过多	*guo duo*	too much
过去	*guo qu*	earlier, formerly
过一个时期	*guo yi ge shi qi*	after a (certain) time
还	*hai*	still, in addition, yet
还故	*hai shi*	still
还褂	*hai you*	there is another...
含有	*han you*	include
好	*hao*	particle indicating the conclusion of the process or activity signified by the immediately preceding verb
好处	*hao chu*	benefit, advantage
好些	*hao xie*	many
和...一样	*he...yi yang*	in the same way as...
合	*he*	together
合并	*he bing*	combine
合乎	*he hu*	conform
合理	*he li*	be appropriate
合适	*he shi*	appropriate
合作	*he zuo*	cooperation
很	*hen*	very
很少	*hen shao*	seldom, rarely
候	*hou*	sign
候测	*hou ce*	assess
后	*hou*	after, behind, latter
后来	*hou lai*	later one
后人	*hou ren*	people in later times

忽地	*hu di*	suddenly, all of a sudden
忽然	*hu ran*	all of a sudden
忽视	*hu shi*	neglect, ignore
互	*hu*	mutual
互相	*hu xiang*	each other, mutually
患	*huan*	suffer (from an illness)
回	*hui*	return
回头	*hui tou*	later on, in a moment
回转	*hui zhuan*	return, turn around
会	*hui*	can be able to
混旌	*hun he*	mix
混焱	*hun tong*	mixed, mixed up, confused
活疃	*huo dong*	activity
其本	*ji ben*	basically, on the whole
其础	*ji chu*	basis
其于	*ji yu*	be based on
其动	*ji dong*	adaptation, flexible, expedient
其会	*ji hui*	opportunity
其能	*ji neng*	function
其转	*ji zhuan*	process
急	*ji*	extremely, exceedingly
急大	*ji da*	very big
急度	*ji du*	extremely, exceedingly
急端	*ji duan*	extreme
急力	*ji li*	by every means possible
急其	*ji qi*	extremely, exceedingly
急速	*ji su*	very fast
及	*ji*	reach, and
及时	*ji shi*	in due time
几	*ji*	some
几个	*ji ge*	some
几十	*ji shi*	tens of...
记录	*ji lu*	record
记录下	*ji lu xia*	record, write down
记诵	*ji song*	learn by heart
记忆力	*ji yi li*	memory
既	*ji*	since
既不...又不	*ji bu...you bu*	neither... nor
既...又	*ji...you*	.... as well as...
继续	*ji xu*	continue
加	*jia*	add
加工	*jia gong*	process

加剧	*jia ju*	increase
加入	*jia ru*	add
加上	*jia shang*	add
加以	*jia yi*	amend by, add
间	*jian*	between, among, in
兼	*jian*	together
兼顾	*jian gu*	take into regard simultaneously
兼施	*jian shi*	apply simultaneously
简单	*jian dan*	simple
简明	*jian ming*	simple and clear
减	*jian*	decrease
减低	*jian di*	reduce
减轻	*jian qing*	alleviate
减小	*jian shao*	lessen, decrease
减退	*jian tui*	decrease
减小	*jian xiao*	decrease
间隔	*jian ge*	interval
间接	*jian jie*	indirect
见	*jian*	appear
见解	*jian jie*	perspective
健康	*jian kang*	health
健全	*jian quan*	be in order, perfect
渐	*jian*	gradually
交	*jiao*	unite
交替	*jiao ti*	alternate
较	*jiao*	relatively, comparatively
叫做	*jiao zuo*	be called, call
接触	*jie chu*	encounter
接近	*jie jin*	be close to
接受	*jie shou*	receive
皆	*jie*	all, both, each and every
阶段	*jie duan*	phase
结实	*jie shi*	firm, stable
结果	*jie guo*	result
结合	*jie he*	link, connect
结论	*jie lun*	conclusion
结束	*jie shu*	finish, be finished
借	*jie*	make use of, borrow
借...来说	*jie...lai shuo*	state in terms of...
今	*jin*	now, today, at present
紧接	*jin jie*	follow, next
仅	*jin*	only, merely, sets a restriction on the quantity
仅是...而已	*jin shi...er yi*	be nothing but...

进入	*jin ru*	enter
进退	*jin tui*	come and go
进行	*jin xing*	conduct, carry on
进一步	*jin yi bu*	in a next step, then
近来	*jin lai*	recently
尽	*jin*	completely
究竟	*jiu jing*	in the end, finally
纠正	*jiu zheng*	correct
久	*jiu*	enduring
就	*jiu*	particle indicating a subsequent process as an obvious consequence of the condition mentioned before
就...来说	*jiu...lai shuo*	take... as example
就是	*jiu shi*	that is
居住	*ju zhu*	reside
拒	*ju*	resist, refuse
据	*ju*	evidence
具	*ju*	have
具备	*ju bei*	have
具体	*ju ti*	concrete, specific
具有	*ju you*	possess, have
俱	*ju*	all, both
剧	*ju*	worsen
剧烈	*ju lie*	violent
觉	*jue*	perceive
绝对	*jue dui*	definitely
均	*jun*	all, both, without exception
均匀	*jun yun*	evenly
开	*kai*	open
开始	*kai shi*	begin
看	*kan*	view
看...来	*kan...lai*	observe (in order) to (do)
看成	*kan cheng*	view as
看出	*kan chu*	recognize
可	*ke*	can, be able, ok
可	*ke hui*	definitely
可考	*ke kao*	certainly
可以	*ke yi*	can, be able
可知	*ke zhi*	it can be realized
客观	*ke guan*	objective
肯定	*ken ding*	confirm
来	*lai*	come, in order to

来往	*lai wang*	come and go
了	*le*	particle defining the immediately preceding verb as past tense
类	*lei*	type, category
类似	*lei si*	resemble
类推	*lei tui*	deduce analogously
类型	*lei xing*	type
离	*li*	leave, defy, go against
理	*li*	principle, theory
理解	*li jie*	understand
理论	*li lun*	theory
理由	*li you*	reason, cause
利用	*li yong*	use, make use of
例	*li*	example
例如	*li ru*	for example, for instance
例证	*li zheng*	example
联系	*lian xi*	relationship
连连	*lian lian*	again and again, in rapid succession
连年	*lian nian*	in successive years, year after year
连日	*lian ri*	for days on end, day after day
连续	*lian xu*	continually, in succession, in a row
良久	*liang jiu*	long time
两	*liang*	both
了解	*liao jie*	understand, find out
列	*lie*	list, enumerate
列入	*lie ru*	assign
列于	*lie yu*	assign
临时	*lin shi*	temporarily
临症	*lin zheng*	clinical
另外	*ling wai*	in addition, moreover, besides
另	*ling yi*	another
另有	*ling you*	in addition there is
流弊	*liu bi*	unwanted effects, drawbacks
流窜	*liu cuan*	flow through
流利	*liu li*	flow
流入	*liu ru*	flow into
流通	*liu tong*	circulate
流行	*liu xing*	flow
录	*lu*	record
陆续	*lu xu*	one after another, in succession, successively
略	*lue*	slightly a little
论	*lun*	determine, discuss, treatise
论定	*lun ding*	definitive statement
论断	*lun duan*	evaluation

漫无	*man wu*	there is absolutely no...
矛盾	*mao dun*	contradiction
没有	*mei you*	does not exist, there is no...
没有意思的	*mei you yi si de*	meaningless
每	*mei*	each, every time
每一	*mei yi*	each, any
每一个	*mei yi ge*	each
门类	*men lei*	category
弥漫	*mi man*	penetrate, fill
密封	*mi feng*	thoroughly close
密切	*mi qie*	close
免得	*mian de*	so as not to
敏感性	*min gan xing*	susceptibility, sensitivity
明白	*ming bai*	understand
明确	*ming que*	make clear, emphasize
名	*ming*	name
名称	*ming cheng*	designation, name
名词	*ming ci*	designation, name, term
名字	*ming zi*	name, designation
目前	*mu qian*	today, at present
哪些	*na xie*	which
哪一	*na yi*	which
乃	*nai*	hence
乃是	*nai shi*	that is, then it is
耐	*nai*	endure
难道	*nan dao*	used in a rhetorical question to make it more emphatic
难怪	*nan guai*	no wonder
呢	*ne*	particle indicating a question that comes in the natural progression of discourse, *e.g.*, so...
内容	*nei rong*	content
能	*neng*	can, be able
能力	*neng li*	ability
宁可	*ning ke*	would rather
弄	*nong*	make, do
配成	*pei cheng*	combine
配合	*pei he*	combination, matching, combine
配伍	*pei wu*	compose
偏	*pian*	one-sided, tending to
凭	*ping*	by means of
颇	*po*	quite, rather, very

颇为	*po wei*	quite, rather, very
普遍	*pu bian*	universal, ubiquitous, general
普通	*pu tong*	general
期	*qi*	phase
其	*qi*	his, her, its
其次	*qi ci*	furthermore, next
其实	*qi shi*	in fact, actually, as a matter of fact
其它	*qi ta*	others
其他	*qi ta*	others
其余	*qi yu*	the remaining
其中	*qi zhong*	among them
奇	*qi*	extraordinary
起	*qi*	bring forth, set off
起来	*qi lai*	raise, mention
起有	*qi you*	fulfill
启发	*qi fa*	enlighten
恰好	*qia hao*	as luck would have it
恰恰	*qia qia*	just right, exactly, precisely
前	*qian*	before, in front of, former
前...后	*qian...hou*	first..., then
前人	*qian ren*	former people, predecessors
且	*qie*	even, and
切忌	*qie ji*	definitely not do or be something
切宜	*qie yi*	it is necessary
轻	*qing*	light, minor
轻减	*qing jian*	lessen
倾向	*qing xiang*	tendency
情况	*qing kuang*	condition
求	*qiu*	search
求得	*qiu de*	find out
趋势	*qu shi*	tend, tendency
区别	*qu bie*	distinguish
取	*qu*	get (something as a result of an investigation), notice, use, take
去	*qu*	go, in order to, remove
去掉	*qu diao*	eliminate
全	*quan*	whole, total
全部	*quan bu*	entirety
全面	*quan mian*	complete, total, entirety
却	*que*	retreat, leave
群	*qun*	group
然	*ran*	like, as if

然而	*ran er*	still, however
然后	*ran hou*	then, afterwards
忍	*ren*	bear, endure
任何	*ren he*	each, any
任何...都	*ren he yi... dou*	everybody, each
认识	*ren shi*	recognize, cognition
认识到	*ren shi dao*	realize, recognize
认为	*ren wei*	deem, think, consider, hold
仍	*reng*	still
仍旧	*reng jiu*	as before, unchanged
仍	*reng ran*	still, yet, nevertheless
日渐	*ri jian*	daily, day by day
日益	*ri yi*	increasingly, increase day by day
容易	*rong yi*	simple
如	*ru*	like, as if
如...便 是	*ru...bian shi*	for example
如果	*ru guo*	if, when
如何	*ru he*	how to
如前所说	*ru qian suo shuo*	as stated before
如同	*ru tong*	same as, as if
入	*ru*	enter
若	*ruo*	if, when
善	*shan*	tend to
善于	*shan yu*	be good for, be suited for
上	*shang*	on, in, over, up
上的	*shang de*	being present in, concerning
上述	*shang shu*	mentioned above
上所述	*shang suo shu*	said above
尚	*shang*	still
少	*shao*	few, little
甚	*shen*	severe, very, greatly
甚至	*shen zhi*	even, possibly going as far as to
生出	*sheng chu*	generate
生活	*sheng huo*	life
生机	*sheng ji*	life process
生理	*sheng li*	physiology
升提	*sheng ti*	rise
失常	*shi chang*	irregular
十分	*shi fen*	very, fully, 100%
失却	*shi que*	miss entirely
时	*shi*	time, while, during
时常	*shi chang*	often, constantly

时候	*shi hou*	time
时间	*shi jian*	time
时期	*shi qi*	period of time
实际	*shi ji*	reality
实际上	*shi ji shang*	in reality
实践	*shi jian*	practice
实验	*shi yan*	experiment, experimental
实有	*shi you*	fact
实质上	*shi zhi shang*	in essence, in reality
识	*shi*	recognize
史	*shi*	history
使	*shi*	cause, if, given
使用	*shi yong*	apply
始	*shi*	begin
势必	*shi bi*	inevitable
适	*shi*	suitable, appropriate
适当	*shi dang*	appropriate
适应	*shi ying*	be suited for
适应范围	*shi ying fan wei*	scope of indications
适用	*shi yong*	suitable
视	*shi*	observe, behold
视...而 定	*shi...er ding*	determine on the basis of
首先	*shou xian*	first
输送	*shu song*	transportation
熟悉	*shu xi*	be familiar with
属	*shu*	belong to, pertain to
属性	*shu xing*	attribute
属于	*shu yu*	be associated with, belong to
数	*shu*	number
数次	*shu ci*	several times, repeatedly
顺便	*shun bian*	in passing
顺从	*shun cong*	go along with
顺手	*shun shou*	in passing, conveniently
说成	*shuo cheng*	designate as, speak of
说法	*shuo fa*	opinion, statement
说明	*shuo ming*	explain
数	*shuo*	frequent, accelerated, fast
思想	*si xiang*	thought idea
四周	*si zhou*	in all four directions, all around
似	*si*	appear like
俟	*si*	wait, only then
俗	*su*	commonly
俗称	*su cheng*	be commonly called

俗呼	*su hu*	be commonly called
素	*su*	permanent, since birth, usually, always, habitually
虽	*sui*	even though, although
虽然	*sui ran*	even though, although
隋	*sui*	follow, afterwards, subsequently
隋处	*sui chu*	everywhere
隋地	*sui di*	anywhere, everywhere
所	*suo*	relative pronoun
所属	*suo shu*	associated with, belonging to
所说的	*suo shuo de*	so-called
所谓	*suo wei*	so-called
所以	*suo yi*	hence, so, therefore, as a result
...所致	*...suo zhi*	be caused by...
他	*ta*	he, she
它	*ta*	it
它的	*ta de*	its
它们	*ta men*	they, them
谈不到	*tan bu dao*	cannot be said, be impossible
探	*tan*	investigate
探求	*tan qiu*	search, investigate
惝...便	*tang...bian*	if..., then
惝...则	*tang...ze*	if..., then
特	*te*	special, exceptional
特别	*te bie*	particular, special, high degree
特长	*te chang*	strength, advantage
特点	*te dian*	characteristic
特殊	*te shu*	specific, special
特易	*te yi*	particularly
特有	*te you*	characteristic, unique
特征	*te zheng*	characteristic
提出	*ti chu*	propose
提高	*ti gao*	increase
体会	*ti hui*	knowledge based on experience
体系	*ti xi*	system
体质	*ti zhi*	physical constitution
体状	*ti zhuang*	physical appearance
条件	*tiao jian*	condition, precondition
通过	*tong guo*	pass through, by way of
同	*tong*	same, similar, identical
同时	*tong shi*	at the same time
同样	*tong yang*	likewise, similarly
同一	*tong yi*	identical

统一	*tong yi*	united, unity
推而至于	*tui er zhi yu*	as for...
推广	*tui guang*	extend
顽固性	*wan gu xing*	stubborn, recalcitrant
完	*wan*	complete, end
完备	*wan bei*	perfect, complete
完全	*wan quan*	complete
完整	*wan zheng*	integrated
挽回	*wan hui*	retrieve
万物	*wan wu*	the tens of thousands of things, all things
万象	*wan xiang*	all phenomena, myriad phenomena
网罗	*wang luo*	interconnect
往来	*wang lai*	come and go
往往	*wang wang*	often
危急	*wei ji*	critical, in severe danger
惟	*wei*	however, only
为	*wei*	be, is
惟持	*wei chi*	maintain
为了	*wei le*	for, on behalf of
未	*wei*	negative in the past, a negative *fait accompli*
未必	*wei bi*	may not
未曾	*wei ceng*	no, not, negative in the past
未尝	*wei chang*	no, not, negative in the past
未...前	*wei...qian*	before...
位置	*wei zhi*	location
谓	*wei*	name, call
紊乱	*wen luan*	disorder
问	*wen*	ask
问题	*wen ti*	issue, question
我	*wo*	I, me
我们	*wo men*	we, us
我们的	*wo men de*	ours
无	*wu*	have not, does not exist, is not
无常	*wu chang*	irregular
无从	*wu cong*	have no basis from which to (do something), not know where to begin
无反	*wu fan*	there is no harm in, might as well
无非	*wu fei*	nothing but, no more than, simply, only
无论	*wu lun*	regardless whether
无数	*wu shu*	innumerable, countless
无所谓	*wu suo wei*	it is impossible to speak of
无以	*wu yi*	have nothing to

物质	*wu zhi*	matter, substance
习贯上	*xi guan shang*	traditionally, usually
系	*xi*	belong to
系列	*xi lie*	series
系统	*xi tong*	system
细致地说	*xi zhi de shuo*	strictly speaking, looked at in detail
狭义	*xia yi*	narrow sense
下	*xia*	down, under, below, descend
先	*xian*	first, for the time being, temporarily
先后	*xian hou*	one after another, successively
先期	*xian qi*	in advance, early, ahead of schedule
衔接	*xian jie*	link
显明	*xian ming*	significant
显示	*xian shi*	show, be a sign of
显箸	*xian zhu*	obvious
现	*xian*	bring forth, cause to appear
现代	*xian dai*	present, modern
现象	*xian xiang*	phenomenon
现在	*xian zhai*	now
相	*xiang*	mutual
相比	*xiang bi*	compare
相成	*xiang cheng*	be mutually complementary
相传	*xiang chuan*	transmit each other
相当	*xiang dang*	quite, fairly, considerable
相得益彰	*xiang de yi zhang*	be of mutual complementarity
相对	*xiang dui*	be mutually opposite
相反	*xiang fan*	be mutually contradictory, on the contrary
相符	*xiang fu*	correspond to each other
相贯	*xiang guan*	linked to each other
相互	*xiang hu*	mutual
相继	*xiang ji*	in succession, one after another
相似	*xiang si*	be similar
相隋	*xiang sui*	follow each other
相提并论	*xiang ti bing lun*	refer to (various things) together
相同	*xiang tong*	identical
详细	*xiang xi*	detailed
想	*xiang*	think of, consider
想必	*xiang bi*	most probably, presumably
向	*xiang*	always, all along
向来	*xiang lai*	always, all along
象	*xiang*	for example
消长	*xiao zhang*	waxing and waning

效	*xiao*	effect
效果	*xiao guo*	result
效能	*xiao neng*	effect
效用	*xiao yong*	effect
些	*xie*	some
协调	*xie tiao*	harmonize, harmony
协助	*xie zhu*	support
挟	*xie*	in conjunction with
新	*xin*	new, just
心理上	*xin li shang*	psychological
形容	*xing rong*	describe
省	*xing*	recognize, know
性能	*xing neng*	ability, effect
性质	*xing zhi*	quality, nature
修	*xiu*	study, care about
需要	*xu yao*	must, need to
须	*xu*	must
须臾	*xu yu*	moment
许多	*xu duo*	many
叙	*xu*	assess
叙述	*xu shu*	discuss, outline
序	*xu*	order
选择	*xuan ze*	select
学术	*xue shu*	science
学说	*xue shuo*	theory, doctrine
学习	*xue xi*	study
循	*xun*	follow
循行	*xun xing*	penetrate, pass through
寻求	*xun qiu*	investigate
迅速	*xun su*	speedy
严重	*yan zhong*	serious
研究	*yan jiu*	research
沿用	*yan yong*	remain in use
样	*yang*	type
要	*yao*	certainly, definitely
要不	*yao bu*	otherwise, or else
要不得	*yao bu de*	no good, intolerable
要不然	*yao bu ran*	otherwise, or else
要不是	*yao bu shi*	if not for
也	*ye*	too, also, either
也就是	*ye jiu shi*	in other words
也许	*ye xu*	perhaps, probably, maybe

一般	*yi ban*	in general, generally
一般的说	*yi ban de shuo*	generally speaking
一道	*yi dao*	together
一点	*yi dian*	not a bit, absolutely not
一定	*yi ding*	definitely, specific
一度	*yi du*	once, for a time in the past
一方面...,方面	*yi fang mian..., fang mian*	on the one hand..., on the other
一概	*yi gai*	one and all, without exception
一共	*yi gong*	in all, altogether, in total
一经	*yi jing*	once, as soon as
一块儿	*yi kuai er*	together
一连	*yi lian*	in succession, continuously, one after another
一起	*yi qi*	together
一切	*yi qie*	all, each
一下	*yi xia*	in an instant, all at once
一向	*yi xiang*	consistently, all along
一些	*yi xie*	some
一样	*yi yang*	in the same way
一再	*yi zai*	again and again
一致	*yi zhi*	identical
一总	*yi zong*	in all, together, in total
依	*yi*	depend on
依...来	*yi...lai*	in accordance with
依次	*yi ci*	in succession, in proper order, one after another
依旧	*yi jiu*	as before
依据	*yi ju*	foundation
依然	*yi ran*	as before
依稀	*yi xi*	vaguely, dimly
已	*yi*	already
已...时,则	*yi...shi, ze...*	if already..., then...
已经	*yi jing*	already
已往	*yi wang*	earlier, in the past
...以后	*...yi hou*	after
以	*yi*	in order to, for, take, by means of
以...来说	*yi...lai shuo*	as far as... is concerned
以...为例	*yi...wei li*	take...as an example
以...为主	*yi...wei zhu*	rest mainly on
以...为...	*yi...wei...*	consider...as...
以便	*yi bian*	in order to, so that, in order to
以及	*yi ji*	as well as, up to
以免	*yi mian*	lest, in order to avoid
以上	*yi shang*	above
以至	*yi zhi*	even, down to, up to

以致	*yi zhi*	as a result, consequently
亦	*yi*	still, also, too, either
意思	*yi si*	meaning
意义	*yi yi*	meaning, significance
异	*yi*	be different
异常	*yi chang*	abnormal
异乎寻常	*yi hu xun chang*	unusual
因	*yin*	follow, because, on account of
因此	*yin ci*	hence
因而	*yin er*	hence
因素	*yin su*	element, factor
因为	*yin wei*	because
引到	*yin dao*	guide
引发	*yin fa*	bring forth
引起	*yin qi*	set off, cause
引用	*yin yong*	apply, make use of
应	*ying*	correspondence, respond, should must
应当	*ying dang*	should, must
应该	*ying gai*	should, must
影响	*ying xiang*	influence
应用	*ying yong*	apply
用	*yong*	employ, use
用…来	*yong…lai*	with
用…作	*yong…zuo…*	use…for
用处	*yong chu*	application
用法	*yong fa*	application
尤	*you*	especially
尤其是	*you qi shi*	especially
尤为	*you wei*	especially
由	*you*	from, take its origin in
由于	*you yu*	because of
有	*you*	have, exist, some
有的	*you de*	some
有关	*you guan*	be related to
有机	*you ji*	organic
有时	*you shi*	sometimes, occasionally
有所	*you suo*	there is something which, a little
有无	*you wu*	whether or not
有限	*you xian*	limited
有效	*you xiao*	effective
有些	*you xie*	there are some, some
有形	*you xing*	tangible
有余	*you yu*	be present in surplus

又	*you*	still, again
又如	*you ru*	as a further example, on the other hand
于	*yu*	at, in
于此可见	*yu ci ke jian*	that shows, from this it can be seen
予	*yu*	give
与	*yu*	and, with
与...相	*yu...xiang*	in comparison to
与...相同	*yu...xiang tong*	identical with
与否	*yu fou*	or not
愈	*yu*	more, even more
愈加	*yu jia*	all the more, even more, furthermore
预	*yu*	in advance, beforehand
预后	*yu hou*	prognosis
预为	*yu wei*	prepare
原是	*yuan shi*	is/are basically
原因	*yuan yin*	cause
原则	*yuan ze*	guiding or basic principle
源	*yuan*	source
约制	*yue zhi*	restrict
匀	*yun*	even
运用	*yun yong*	apply
杂	*za*	various, mixed, miscellaneous
哉	*zai*	particle emphasizing the preceding statement
再	*zai*	again
再次	*zai ci*	still another
再说	*zai shuo*	what's more, moreover
在	*zai*	in, at, be there, exist, particle indicating the continuous form of the subsequent verb
在...的	*zai...de*	being in
在...方面	*zai...fang mian*	as for
在...上	*zai...shang*	in..., as for
在...时	*zai...shi*	while, during
在...时候	*zai...shi hou*	while, during
在...下	*zai...xia*	under
在...中	*zai...zhong*	within
在...中的	*zai...zhong de*	being present in
在于	*zai yu*	be in, take place in
造成	*zao cheng*	bring forth
则	*ze*	then
增加	*zeng jia*	increase
占	*zhan*	assume (a stage)
占有	*zhan you*	have

着	*zhao*	reach, get to, press against
找到	*zhao dao*	find out
找寻	*zhao xun*	search
照理	*zhao li*	logically, morally
照例	*zhao li*	as a rule, as usual
照说	*zhao shuo*	logically, morally
折	*zhe*	break
者	*zhe*	particle defining the immediately preceding verb or number as a noun referring to an item or a person
这	*zhe*	this, these
这就	*zhe jiu*	that is
这类	*zhe lei*	such
这里	*zhe li*	here
这些	*zhe xie*	these
这样	*zhe yang*	such
这	*zhe yi*	this
这种	*zhe zhong*	this
着	*zhe*	particle defining the immediately preceding verb as a gerund
真	*zhen*	really, truly, indeed
征象	*zheng xiang*	sign
整个	*zheng ge*	entire
整套	*zheng tao*	complete system, set
整体	*zheng ti*	whole
正	*zheng*	proper, normal, regular, correct, a particle indicating an action in progress
正常	*zheng chang*	normal
正在	*zheng zai*	be just (in a specific state)
症候	*zheng hou*	symptoms
症象	*zheng xiang*	sign
证明	*zheng ming*	demonstrate
证实	*zheng shi*	evidence
之	*zhi*	this, particle identifying the immediately preceding expression as a possessive
之后	*zhi hou*	following, after
之间	*zhi jian*	among, between
之外	*zhi wai*	in addition to
之一	*zhi yi*	one of
职司	*zhi si*	regulate, manage
直	*zhi*	straight, upright, lengthwise, direct, continuously
直接	*zhi jie*	direct
只	*zhi*	only
只顾	*zhi gu*	merely, simply, be absorbed in
只管	*zhi guan*	merely, simply, be absorbed in

只是	*zhi shi*	it is just that
只要	*zhi yao*	all that is necessary is, as long as, provided that
只有	*zhi you*	only if, only when
至	*zhi*	arrive, reach
至...为度	*zhi...wei du*	until...
至...为止	*zhi...wei zhi*	until...
至多	*zhi duo*	at most
至少	*zhi shao*	at least
至于	*zhi yu*	as for, as far as, to such an extent as to
置	*zhi*	bring, put
制成	*zhi cheng*	prepare
制法	*zhi fa*	production method
中	*zhong*	center, amidst, in, among
中间	*zhong jian*	be between
终身	*zhong shen*	the entire life
种	*zhong*	type, measure word for abstract concepts
种类	*zhong lei*	kind, type
重大	*zhong da*	important
重量	*zhong liang*	weight
重视	*zhong shi*	regard highly, pay attention to
重要	*zhong yao*	important
重要性	*zhong yao xing*	importance
众	*zhong*	numerous
诸	*zhu*	all
逐步	*zhu bu*	step by step, gradually
逐渐	*zhu jian*	slowly, gradually
逐	*zhu yi*	one by one
主持	*zhu chi*	direct, be responsible for
主司	*zhu si*	be responsible for
主要	*zhu yao*	main, basically, in principle
注	*zhu*	comment
注解	*zhu jie*	comment
注意	*zhu yi*	pay attention
抓住	*zhua zhu*	get hold of
专	*zhuan*	only, exclusively
专门	*zhuan men*	exclusively, specialized
专	*zhuan yi*	concentrated
专为	*zhuan wei*	change into
转	*zhuan*	turn around
状	*zhuang*	appearance
准保	*zhun bao*	certainly, for sure
准确	*zhun que*	real, realistic
准则	*zhun ze*	criterion

着实	*zhuo shi*	truly, really
着重	*zhuo zhong*	emphasize, stress
兹	*zi*	here, now
资生	*zi sheng*	create
资态	*zi tai*	posture
仔细	*zi xi*	carefully
自	*zi*	from, self, of course, automatic, spontaneous
自己	*zi ji*	self, own
自觉	*zi jue*	subjective
自然	*zi ran*	nature, natural
自然界	*zi ran jie*	the natural world, nature
自主	*zi zhu*	self-control
字	*zi*	a Chinese character
综合	*zong he*	comprehensive
总	*zong*	always, invariably
总的说来	*zong de shuo lai*	generally speaking
总共	*zong gong*	in all, altogether
总括	*zong kuo*	survey
总时	*zong shi*	always, invariably
总算	*zong suan*	at long last
总之	*zong zhi*	in general, to sum up, in a word
走	*zou*	go, move
最	*zui*	very, extreme
最多	*zui duo*	at most
最好	*zui hao*	had better, it would be better
最后	*zui hou*	very last
最少	*zui shao*	at least
最为	*zui wei*	be the most...
最早	*zui zao*	earliest
尊为	*zun wei*	revere as
佐	*zuo*	assist
作	*zuo*	make, serve as
作成	*zuo cheng*	form to...
作出	*zuo chu*	produce, generate
作为	*zuo wei*	consider as
作业	*zuo ye*	work
作用	*zuo yong*	function, effect

18
Looking Up Complicated Characters

As mentioned above, the most commonly used and available Chinese-English dictionary for looking up complicated or traditional, unsimplified characters is *Mathew's Chinese English Dictionary*. Unlike Pinyin Chinese-English dictionaries based on PRC models, *Mathews's* list of radicals is found in the back on page 1179 as Appendix B. Two hundred fourteen radicals are listed on this page and the next. They are presented in terms of the number of strokes with which they are written. However, because some of the radicals have themselves been simplified, these radicals do not all carry the same number of strokes and, therefore, the same numerical identification as do the radicals in your Pinyin Chinese-English dictionary. Below is a reproduction of *Mathew's* radical index.

THE 214 RADICALS.

N B.—The numbers in the Dictionary under which the Radicals occur may be ascertained from the Radical Index.   The more common Radicals are printed in large type.   Such abbreviated forms as, e. g., Nos. 9, 18, etc., do not usually stand alone, but are found in combination only.

No.	Radical	No.	Radical	No.	Radical	No.	Radical	No.	Radical
Strokes		23	匸	46	山	68	斗	92	牙
1		24	十	47	巛川巜	69	斤	93	牛牜
1	一	25	卜	48	工	70	方	94	犬犭
2	丨	26	卩㔾	49	己	71	无旡		
3	丶	27	厂	50	巾	72	日	**5**	
4	丿	28	厶	51	干	73	曰	95	玄
5	乙	29	又	52	幺	74	月	96	玉王王
6	亅			53	广	75	木	97	瓜
2		**3**		54	廴	76	欠	98	瓦
7	二	30	口	55	廾	77	止	99	甘
8	亠	31	囗	56	弋	78	歹歺	100	生
9	人亻	32	土	57	弓	79	殳	101	用
10	儿	33	士	58	彐彑	80	毋	102	田
11	入	34	夂	59	彡	81	比	103	疋
12	八	35	夊	60	彳	82	毛	104	疒
13	冂	36	夕			83	氏	105	癶
14	冖	37	大	**4**		84	气	106	白
15	冫	38	女	61	心忄小	85	水氵	107	皮
16	几	39	子	62	戈	86	火灬	108	皿
17	凵	40	宀	63	戶	87	爪爫	109	目罒
18	刀刂	41	寸	64	手才	88	父	110	矛
19	力	42	小	65	支	89	爻	111	矢
20	勹	43	尢兀尣	66	攴攵	90	爿	112	石
21	匕	44	尸	67	文	91	片	113	示礻
22	匚	45	屮					114	禸

No.	Radical
115	禾
116	穴
117	立
6	
118	竹⺮
119	米
120	糸糹
121	缶
122	网罒罓
123	羊
124	羽
125	老
126	而
127	耒
128	耳
129	聿
130	肉月
131	臣
132	自
133	至
134	臼
135	舌
136	舛
137	舟

(1179)

APPENDIX B. RADICALS. (Continued).

138 艮	152 豕	**8**	181 頁	**11**	207 鼓
139 色	153 豸	167 金	182 風	195 魚	208 鼠
140 艸 艹	154 貝	168 長 镸	183 飛	196 鳥	**14**
141 虍	155 赤	169 門	184 食	197 鹵	209 鼻
142 虫	156 走	170 阜 阝	185 首	198 鹿	210 齊
143 血	157 足	171 隶	186 香	199 麥	**15**
144 行	158 身	172 隹	**10**	200 麻	211 齒
145 衣 衤	159 車	173 雨 ⻗	187 馬	**12**	**16**
146 西	160 辛	174 青	188 骨	201 黃	212 龍
7	161 辰	175 非	189 高	202 黍	213 龜
147 見	162 辵 辶	**9**	190 髟	203 黑	**17**
148 角	163 邑 阝	176 面	191 鬥	204 黹	214 龠
149 言	164 酉	177 革	192 鬯	**13**	
150 谷	165 釆	178 韋	193 鬲	205 黽	
151 豆	166 里	179 韭	194 鬼	206 鼎	
		180 音			

Once you have found the number of the radical of the character you are trying to look up, then you turn to the radical in what *Mathew's* calls its Radical Index. Actually, this is corresponds to the Character Index in our Pinyin Chinese-English dictionary. Turn to the page on which the number of the radical of your character begins (1181). The radical number is written in Arabic numerals and is centered on the column with a horizontal line drawn under it. Then search down the columns under the numbers of strokes. The numbers of strokes are written in Arabic numerals and are placed on the left-hand sides of the columns. Remember that you are only counting the number of the remaining strokes minus the radical. When you find the character you are looking for, you will see that there is an Arabic numeral on the right-hand side of the column. This is the page number on which the character is found. Now turn to that page and scan for the bold-faced, larger character which you are trying to find.

This process is basically identical to looking up characters in your Pinyin Chinese-English dictionary. The only differences are that the radical and character indexes are located at the rear of *Matnew's*, that the radicals are differently numbered and some have more strokes, and that the romanization of the pronunciation of the characters is given in Wade-Giles system rather than in Pinyin. In Appendix 1, I give conversions for the Pinyin, Wade-Giles, and Yale systems of romanization, the three main systems of romanization of Chinese in use today.

A Quick Cross-reference of Simplified & Complex Characters

At the back of your Pinyin Chinese-English dictionary, after the last definition, you should find an appendix (附录, *fu lu*) titled, "The Original Complex Forms of Chinese Characters and Their

Simplified Versions." This chart is alphabetized in terms of Pinyin spelling. The simplified forms of the characters are given on the left followed by the complex forms in brackets on the right. This chart can really only help you look up a complex character if you already A) have a hunch what it stands for and B) know the word's Pinyin spelling. In that case, you can scan the list of characters under the first letter of the word's Pinyin spelling and check to see if the complex form is given next to simplified character you thought. Frankly, this is not a hugely useful appendix. It is only really useful for those who have learned the simplified characters, know their Pinyin romanization, and want to know how to write a particular character in its complex form. This is not a skill commonly called upon when translating.

19
Special Problems in Identifying Chinese Medicinals

As you will quickly come to realize, the Chinese medical literature primarily deals with so-called herbal medicine. Therefore, if you do much translating of the Chinese medical literature and do not confine yourself specifically to subspecialties like acupuncture, dietary therapy, *tui na*, or *qi gong*, you will eventually face certain problems with identifying Chinese medicinals.

In Chapter 14, I have given a list of 403 Chinese medicinals. This list will stand you in good stead in most cases. However, every now and again, you will come across a medicinal which is not on this list or not in Bensky & Gamble's *Chinese Herbal Medicine: Materia Medica*. Bensky & Gamble is the most commonly used Chinese materia medica at American colleges of Chinese medicine. Although it is an excellent book in terms of the basic information given on each individual medicinal, the number of medicinals it contains is not sufficient once you start seriously translating. So what to do?

In my experience, the single best way to identify a Chinese medicinal which is not in Bensky & Gamble is to look it up in the 中药大词典 (*Zhong Yao Da Ci Dian*). We already know that *zhong yao* means Chinese medicinals. *Da* means great or large. *Ci dian* means dictionary. Therefore, *Zhong Yao Da Ci Dian* means *The Large Dictionary of Chinese Medicinals*. This dictionary contains more than 5,700 Chinese medicinals, and is one of the best references for finding obscure Chinese medicinals. (It also contains much more information about each medicinal than does Bensky & Gamble as we will see below.)

The *Zhong Yao Da Ci Dian* comes in two volumes. 上 (*shang*) means upper, but, in terms of a multi-volume set of books, means Vol. 1. 下 (*xia*) means lower, but here means Vol. 2. (If there were a third volume, Vol. 2 would be labeled 中 (*zhong*, middle), while Vol. 3 would be labeled 下 (*xia*). On page number 1 of Vol. 1, you will find the medicinal index for that volume. Vol. 1 contains all those medicinals the first character of whose names are written with from one to eight strokes. Vol. 2 contains all those medicinals whose first characters contain nine or more strokes. To use this table of contents or medicinal index, you simply count the *total number of strokes* of the first character in the medicinal's name. Like your Pinyin Chinese-English dictionary, this medicinal index uses Chinese numbers for the stroke number headings. Below is a reproduction of the first page of Vol. 1 showing the listings for medicinals whose first characters contain one, two, or three strokes. (The three stroke characters continue on the succeeding pages.)

目　录

（一至八画）

Having found the column of characters under the number of strokes of the first character in the medicinal's name, you must scan down this column until you find the first character. Then you must scan all the medicinals whose names begin with this character until you find a match for the second (and possibly third or fourth characters of the name). For instance, you are looking for the medicinal whose name is written 丁香 (*Ding Xiang*). The character *ding* is written with two strokes. So we scan down the column of two stroke first characters. Once we find *ding*, we see that there are 10 medicinals all of whose names begin with the character *ding*. However, in this case, our search is easy. There is only one medicinal listed whose name begins with *ding* and is only two characters long. To the left of *Ding Xiang*, we find the number 0026. This means that *ding xiang* is the 26th medicinal discussed in this dictionary. To the right of *Ding Xiang*, we find the number 13. This means that *Ding Xiang*'s discussion begins on page 13.

热，头晕耳鸣，腰酸腿软，心烦，目赤。
①《本草再新》："治虚劳咳嗽。"
②《植物名实图考》："治吐血。"
③《饮片新参》："治肺劳，止咳化痰，退虚热，杀虫。"
④《现代实用中药》："清凉性滋养强壮药。功效与女贞子相似，适用于潮热、骨蒸、腰酸、膝软、头晕、耳鸣等证。"
⑤《陆川本草》："泻火退热。治温病发热，心烦，下利，赤眼。"
⑥《西藏常用中草药》："治湿热痢疾，目赤肿痛，痈肿疮毒。"
【用法与用量】 内服：煎汤，2～3钱
【选方】 治风火牙痛：十大功劳叶三钱，水煎顿服，每日一剂，痛甚者服二剂。(《江西草药》)
【备考】 《植物名实图考》："十大功劳，生广信。丛生，硬茎直黑，对叶排比，光泽而劲，锯齿如刺，梢端生长须数茎，结小实似鱼子兰。""又一种，叶细长，齿短无刺，开花成簇，亦如鱼子兰。"

0026 **丁香** dīng xiāng （《药性论》）

【异名】 丁子香(《齐民要术》)，支解香、雄丁香(《本草蒙筌》)，公丁香(《本草原始》)。
【基源】 为桃金娘科植物丁香的花蕾。
【原植物】 丁香 *Syzygium aromaticum* (L.) Merr. et Perry
常绿乔木，高达10米。叶对生；叶柄明显；叶片长方卵形或长方倒卵形，长5～10厘米，宽2.5～5厘米，先端渐尖或急尖，基部狭窄常下展成柄，全缘，花芳香，成顶生聚伞圆锥花序，花径约6毫米；花萼肥厚，绿色后转紫色，长管状，先端4裂，裂片三角形；花冠白色，稍带淡紫，短管状，4裂；雄蕊多数，花药纵裂；子房下位，与萼管合生，花柱粗肥，柱头不明显。浆果红棕色，长方椭圆形，长1～1.5厘米，直径5～8毫米，先端宿存萼片。种子长方形。
分布马来群岛及非洲，我国广东、广西等地有栽培。
本植物的树根（丁香根）、树皮（丁香树皮）、树枝（丁香枝）、果实（母丁香）、花蕾蒸馏所得的挥发油（丁香油）亦供药用，各详专条。
【采集】 通常在9月至次年3月间，花蕾由青转为鲜红色时采收。采下后除去花梗，晒干。
【药材】 干燥的花蕾略呈短棒状，长1.5～2厘米，红棕色至暗棕色。下部为圆柱状略扁的萼管，长1～1.3厘米，宽约5毫米，厚约3毫米，基部渐狭小，表面粗糙，刻之有油渗出，萼管上端有4片三角形肥厚的萼。上部近圆球形，径约6毫米，具花瓣4片，互相抱合。将花蕾

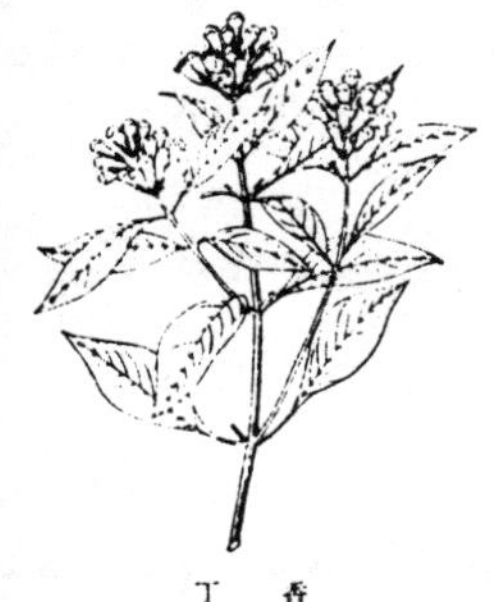

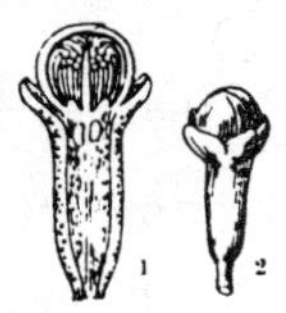

丁香
1.花蕾纵切面 2.花蕾

剖开，可见多数雄蕊，花丝向中心弯曲，中央有一粗壮直立的花柱。质坚实而重，入水即沉；断面有油性，用指甲划之可见油质渗出。气强烈芳香，味辛。以个大、粗壮、鲜紫棕色、香气强烈、油多者为佳。
主产于坦桑尼亚、马来西亚、印度尼西亚等地。我国广东有少数出产。
【成分】 花蕾含挥发油即丁香油。油中主要含有丁香油酚(Eugenol)、乙酰丁香油酚、β-石竹烯(β-Caryophyllene)，以及甲基正戊基酮、水杨酸甲酯、葎草烯(Humulene)、苯甲醛、苄醇、间甲氧基苯甲醛、乙酸苄酯、胡椒酚(Chavicol)、α-衣兰烯(α-Ylangene)等[1]。也有野生品种中不含丁香油酚（平常丁香油中含64～85%），而含丁香酮(Eugenone)和番樱桃素(Eugenin)[2]。花中还含三萜化合物如齐墩果酸(Oleanolic acid)[3]、黄酮和对氧萘酮类鼠李素(Rhamnetin)、山柰酚(Kaempferol)[4]、番樱桃素、番樱桃素亭(Eugenitin)、异番樱桃素亭(Isoeugenitin)及其去甲基化合物异番樱桃酚(Isoeugenitol)[4~7]。
【药理】 ①抗菌作用 含有1%浓度的丁香的乙醚浸出液，水浸液或含8%浓度的丁香煎剂的沙伯氏培养基，对许兰氏黄癣菌、白色念珠菌等多种致病性真菌均有抑制作用[1~2]。较高浓度时对新型隐球菌也有抑制作用[3]。醇浸出液与醚浸出液相似，但水浸液较差[3]。丁香油及丁香油酚在1:8000～1:16000时，对致病性真菌即有抑制作用[4]。煎剂1:20～1:640浓度时，对葡萄球菌、链球菌及白喉、变形、绿脓、大肠、痢疾、伤寒等杆菌均有抑制作用[5~7]。丁香油和丁香油酚在1:2000～1:8000浓度时，对金黄色葡萄球菌及肺炎、痢疾(志贺氏)、大肠、变形、结核菌均有抑菌作用[8,9]。丁香对流感病毒PR8株也有抑制作用（体外试验）[10]。
②驱虫作用 水或醇提取液在体外对猪蛔虫有麻痹或杀死作用，感染蛔虫的狗口服丁香0.5～1.0克/公斤，有驱虫作用，但一次服用并不能将蛔虫全部驱除。丁香油较煎剂为优[11]。
③健胃作用 丁香为芳香健胃剂，可缓解腹部气胀、增强消化能力、减轻恶心呕吐[11]。5%丁香油酚乳剂可使胃粘液分泌显著增加，而酸度则不增强；丁香油之作用稍差，连续应用，可使粘液旺盛，而仅分泌非粘液性的渗出物；36小时后方能部分恢复反应（分泌粘液），完全恢复，需数月以后[13,14]。
④止牙痛 丁香油（少量滴入）可消毒龋齿腔，破坏其神经，从而减轻牙痛[14]。
⑤其他作用 家兔静脉注射丁香油酚，可产生麻醉、降低血压、呼吸抑制与抗惊厥作用。但对小鼠皮下注射，不能产生麻醉作用[14]。丁香还含有子宫收缩成分，易溶于水和乙醇，不易溶于醚、石油醚、氯仿、苯和醋酸[14]。
毒性 小鼠腹腔注射煎剂的半数致死量为1.8克/公斤，口服丁香油的花生油溶液为1.6克/公斤，鱼的中毒症状为呼吸抑制及后肢无力。狗口服丁香油的花生油溶液5克/公斤，可发生呕吐而死亡。尸检发现胃底及幽门部粘膜红肿并有溃疡及出血点，十二指肠部有浮肿及充血，肺有瘀血点，镜检肝、肾也有瘀血及浮肿，部分肝细胞坏死，心肌浊肿。狗如口服2克/公斤，仅发生呕吐而不致死亡[11]。大鼠口服丁香油酚，半数致死量为1.93克/公斤，中毒症状为后肢麻痹、惊厥、尿失禁并常有血尿，病理解剖发见上消化道呈出血状态，少数有粘膜溃疡，各内脏及腹膜、肠系膜缺

Turning to page 13, we find the small uppercase numerals 0026 on the far left column with large, bold-faced 丁香 (*Ding Xiang*). To the right of the Chinese characters, we find the upper case Pinyin, *ding xiang*. Under this name, the first bold-faced characters in brackets say 异名(*Yi ming*), other names. This tells us the other names this medicinal commonly goes by. Next come the bold-faced two characters in brackets which say 基源 (*Ji yuan*), basic source. This then tells us that the part used in medicine is the 花 (*Hua*) 蕾 (*Lei*), flower bud. Under this, there are the bold-faced characters in brackets which say 源植物 (*Yuan zhi wu*). *Yuan* means "source" and *zhi wu* means "plant or flora". So this heading means "the source plant". This is followed by the italicized Linnean binomial nomenclature, *Syzygium aromaticum.* Underneath this is a text-dense botanical description of the clove plant.

(Before going on, the reader should note that the Latinate name Bensky & Gamble give this medicinal is Flos Caryophylli. Flos means flower. Why Bensky & Gamble chose Caryophyllum instead of Syzygium, I don't know. Flos Caryophylli is the Latinate pharmaceutical nomenclature for the part or piece used. Below are some Latin terms used in this pharmaceutical nomenclature that may help you in crafting medicinal identifications in your translations.

Semen = seed
Fructus = fruit
Ramulus = branch or twig
Caulis = vine
Radix = root
Rhizoma = rhizome
Tuber = tuber
Folium = leaf
Flos = flower
Pericarpium = surrounding skin
Exocarpium = outer skin
Cortex = bark

Spica = spike
Spora = spore
Pediculus = pedicle
Os = bone
Cornu = horn
Resina = resin
Gelatinum = gelatin
Concha = shell
Et = and
Seu = or
Cum = with

When using this pharmaceutical nomenclature, the name of the part or piece comes first and is written in nominative case. Then the name of the plant or species comes next. Since the name as a whole says that it is the part or piece *of* such-and-such a plant or animal, the species name is written in genitive or possessive case. Therefore, when following Flos, Caryophyllum becomes Caryophylli. Based on the identification in the *Zhong Yao Da Ci Dian*, we can also identify this medicinal as Flos Syzygii Aromatici.)

Under the botanical description of the clove plant, comes the bold-faced bracketed characters 采集 (*cai ji*). This means to gather or collect. The information given after this heading tells when and how to collect this medicinal. Next comes the bold-faced, bracketed characters 药材 (*yao cai*), crude medicinals. This section tells us about the part or piece being used as the medicinal in question. Under this is the bold-faced, bracketed section headed by the characters 成分 (*cheng fen*), composition. It tells us about the chemical constituents of this medicinal. This is followed by the heading 药理 (*yao li*), pharmacodynamics or pharmacology — difficult to read, Western scientific vocabulary. Under that, the next heading is 毒性 (*du xing*), toxicity. Good information, but very technical. Let's turn the page.

著充血。对中毒大鼠曾用印防己毒素、可拉明、士的宁、咖啡因及五甲烯四氮唑等解救，但无明显效果[11]。

【性味】 辛，温。

①《开宝本草》："味辛，温，无毒。"

②《纲目》："辛，热。"

【归经】 入胃、脾、肾经。

①《汤液本草》："入手太阴、足阳明、少阴经。"

②《雷公炮制药性解》："入肺、脾、胃、肾四经。"

【功用主治】 温中，暖胃，降逆。治呃逆，呕吐，反胃，泻痢，心腹冷痛，痃癖，疝气，癣疾。

①《药性论》："治冷气腹痛。"

②《海药本草》："主风疳匶，骨槽劳臭。治气，乌髭发，杀虫，疗五痔，辟恶去邪。治奶头花，止五色毒痢，正气，止心腹痛。"

③《日华子本草》："治口气，反胃，疗肾气，奔豚气，阴痛，壮阳，暖腰膝，杀酒毒，消痃癖，除冷劳。"

④《开宝本草》："温脾胃，止霍乱。(治)壅胀，风毒诸肿，齿疳匶。"

⑤《本草蒙筌》："止气忒、气逆。"

⑥《纲目》："治虚哕，小儿吐泻，痘疮胃虚灰白不发。"

⑦《本草正》："温中快气。治上焦呃逆，除胃寒泻痢，七情五郁。"

⑧《本草汇》："疗胸痹、阴痛，暖阴户。"

⑨《医林纂要》："补肝、润命门、暖胃、去中寒，泻肺、散风湿。"

⑩《本草再新》："开九窍，舒郁气，去风，行水。"

⑪《药材学》："治慢性消化不良，胃肠充气及子宫疝痛。"

【用法与用量】 内服，煎汤，0.3～1钱；或入丸、散。外用：研末调敷。

【宜忌】 热病及阴虚内热者忌服。

①《雷公炮炙论》："不可见火。畏郁金。"

②李杲："气血胜者不可服，丁香益其气也。"

③《本草经疏》："一切有火热证者忌之，非属虚寒，概勿施用。"

【选方】 ①治伤寒咳噫不止，及哕逆不定：丁香一两，干柿蒂一两。焙干，捣罗为散。每服一钱，煎人参汤下，无时服。(《简要济众方》)

②治小儿吐逆：丁香、半夏(生用)各一两。同研为细末，姜汁和丸，如绿豆大。姜汤下三、二十丸。(《百一选方》)

③治朝食暮吐：丁香十五个研末，甘蔗汁、姜汁和丸莲子大，噙咽之。(《摘元方》)

④治霍乱，止吐：丁香十四枚，以酒五合，煮取二合，顿服之。用水煮之亦佳。(《千金翼方》)

⑤治久心痛不止：丁香半两，桂心一两。捣细，罗为散，每于食前，以热酒调下一钱。(《圣惠方》)

⑥治痈疽恶肉：丁香末敷之，外用膏药护之。(《怪证奇方》)

⑦治食蟹致伤：丁香末，姜汤服五分。(《证治要诀》)

⑧治鼻中息肉：丁香绵裹纳之。(《圣惠方》)

【临床报道】 治癣。丁香15克，加入70%酒精至100毫升，浸48小时后去渣。每日外搽患处3次，观察31例病史在2年以上的体癣及足癣患者，一般在治疗1天后症状即见消退，2天后患处开始有皮屑脱落。病史较长或曾经其它癣药治疗而不能控制者，则于治疗后2～3天症状才开始消退，一般经3～5天亦能治愈。但有20%左右治愈后仍反复发作[1]。一法用1:10的丁香煎液外涂，每日1～3次，治疗数种皮肤霉菌病共31例，结果8例临床痊愈，10例显效，8例有效，5例无效。有效病例通常在涂药后3～7日痒感减轻，炎症减退，落屑减少，以后局部症状逐渐好转。治疗期中如中断用药，效果多不明显或无效。疗效与病原菌未见明显关系。曾对6例治愈患者进行短期随访，1例于1个月后复发，5例经2～12月观察未见复发[2]。

【各家论述】 ①《本草经疏》："丁香，其主温脾胃、止霍乱壅胀者，盖脾胃为仓廪之官，饮食生冷，伤于脾胃，留而不去，则为壅塞胀满，上涌下泄，则为挥霍撩乱，辛温暖脾胃而行滞气，则霍乱止而壅胀消矣。齿疳匶者，亦阳明湿热上攻也，散阳明之邪，则疳匶自除。疗风毒诸肿者，辛温散结，而香气又能走窍除秽浊也。"

②《本草通玄》："丁香，温中健胃，须于丸剂中同润药用乃佳。独用多用，易于僭上，损肺伤目。"

③《本草新编》："丁香，有雌雄之分，其实治病无分彼此。直中阴经之病，最宜用之，但不可用之于传经之伤寒也。"

④《得配本草》："丁香，得五味子治奔豚，配甘蔗、姜汁治干呕。肉桂温能发表，丁香温能和胃。"

【备考】 ①《雷公炮炙论》："凡使(丁香)，有雌雄，雄颗小，雌颗大，似枣核。方中多使雌，力大，膏煎中用雄。"

②《开宝本草》："丁香，二月、八月采。按广州送丁香图，树高丈余，叶似栎叶，花圆细，黄色，凌冬不雕。医家所用惟用根。子如钉子，长三、四分，紫色，中有粗大如山茱萸者，俗呼为母丁香，可入心腹之药尔。"

0027 丁公藤 dīng gōng téng (广州空军《常用中草药手册》)

【异名】 包公藤(广州空军《常用中草药手册》)。

【基原】 为旋花科植物丁公藤的根、茎。

【原植物】 丁公藤 *Erycibe obtusifolia* Benth.

攀缘木质藤本，幼枝被柔毛。单叶互生，椭圆形或倒卵形，长5～9厘米，宽2～5厘米，全缘。聚伞花序，集成圆锥花序，腋生或顶生，花小，金黄色；花冠阔钟形，5深裂；子房1室；浆果球形。种子1颗。

生于疏林或密林中，攀援于树上。分布广东、广西、云南。

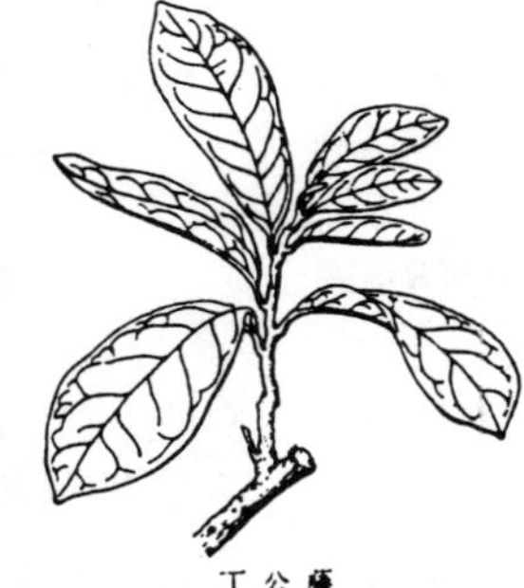

丁公藤

【采集】 全年可采，洗净切成段，隔水蒸2～4小时，晒干备用。

【性味】 广州空军《常用中草药手册》："辛，温，有毒。"

【功用主治】 广州空军《常用中草药手册》："解表发汗，驱风湿，除痹痛，消肿止痛。治风湿痹痛，半身不遂，跌打肿痛。"

【用法与用量】 内服：煎汤，1～2钱；或浸酒。外用：浸酒外搽。

【宜忌】 本品有毒，孕妇忌服。

【临床报道】 治疗风湿背痛及神经痛。丁公藤制成注射液，每支2毫升，含原生药5克，每次2～4毫升，每天1～

Now we see the bold-faced, bracketed heading 性味 (*xing wei*), nature and flavor(s). Nature here means "temperature", while *wei* means "flavors". Next to this heading, you will see the characters 辛(*xin*), acrid, and 温 (*wen*), warm. Under this there are two numbers in circles. After each number, there are a pair of double chevrons with characters inside. These are book titles. For instance, the second one is 纲目 (*Gang Mu*), the abbreviation of Li Shi-zhen's monumental 本草 纲目 (*Ben Cao Gang Mu, Great Outline of the Materia Medica*). These give different opinions about this medicinal's nature and flavor and specifies the cite or source for each opinion. The first listing, which tallies with Bensky & Gamble's, is the current standard opinion in the PRC, but it is good to know that there are other, potentially valid opinions.

Likewise, under the next heading, 归经 (*gui jing*), channel gathering, there is the standard, contemporary opinion and then cites from two premodern sources. Under 功用主治 (*gong yong zhu zhi*, functions and indications, (literally *zhu zhi* means "mainly treats")), there is the standard rap and then cites from 11 different literary sources. Then we have the heading 用法与用... *yong fa yu yong chong*). This means "method of use and amount of use or dosage". Next we have the heading 宣忌 (*xuan ji*), appropriate prohibitions or contraindications. This is followed by the heading 选方 (*xuan fang*), a selection of formulas (all containing this medicinal as a ruling or main ingredient. After that, the next heading says 临床报道 (*lin chuang bao dao*), clinical reports. The next to the last heading says 名家论述 (*ming jia lun shu*), various schools discussions (of this medicinal) with more literary cites on varying points of view. And finally, the last heading says 备考 (*bei kao*), for reference, *i.e.*, an appendix or notes for reference. If you're like me, there's lots of good information waiting here to be translated!

Other useful sources

Personally, I find the *Zhong Yao Da Ci Dian* my single best source for finding problematic Chinese medicinals. However, if you look up the Pinyin spelling of the characters in the name of the medicinal in question, you can also scan the Pinyin index of Hong-yen Hsu's *Oriental Materia Medica: A Concise Guide*. Although the information on each individual medicinal is inferior to the information given in Bensky & Gamble, Hsu's materia medica does include approximately 200 more medicinals. It gives the names of these medicinals in both Pinyin and Wade-Giles as well as complicated and simplified characters. Unfortunately, the Pinyin index is not as complete as the Wade-Giles index, and there are some omissions.

Then there is the six volume set, *Chinese Materia Medica,* published in Taiwan by Southern Materials Center, Inc. One volume is on vegetable medicinals, another is on insect, snake, and fish medicinals, a third is on animal medicinals, the fourth deals with turtles, shellfish, and birds, the fifth deals with famine foods, and the sixth is a botanical, chemical, pharmacological, and reference list for the medicinals in the *Ben Cao Gang Mu (Great Outline of Materia Medica)* mentioned above. Although this set of books was done around the turn of the century and its design and type styles are dated, under each medicinal, it gives a list of alternative names. The characters are the complicated characters and the romanization is Wade-Giles, but many is the time I have found the identification of some obscure alternate name in one of these books.

And a final excellent source for finding alternative medicinal names is the old *A Barefoot*

Doctor's Manual. Under most of the medicinals in this book, there are very complete listings of all the local or regional alternative names of medicinals. The romanization is Wade-Giles, the characters are the complicated ones, and the writing is quite small, but this source should not be left unconsulted before you give up on identifying some trying medicinal.

Alternate names & abbreviations

Many medicinals have more than a single name. For instance, Semen Coicis Lachryma-jobi may be 薏苡仁 (*Yi Yi Ren*), 薏米 (*Yi Mi*), 薏仁 (*Yi Ren*), or 薏米仁 (*Yi Mi Ren*). Radix Scrophulariae Ningpoensis may be either 玄渗 (*Xuan Shen*) or 元渗 (*Yuan Shen*). Radix Morindae Officinalis may be either 巴戟天 (*Ba Ji Tian*) or 巴戟肉 (*Ba Ji Rou*). Fructus Corni Officinalis may be either 山萸萸 (*Shan Zhu Yu*), 山萸肉 (*Shan Yu Rou*), or 山萸肉 (*Shan Zhu Rou*). Arillus Euphoriae Longanae may be either 龙眼肉 (*Long Yan Rou*) or 桂元肉 (*Gui Yuan Rou*). And Rhizoma Corydalis Yanhusuo may be 延胡索 (*Yan Hu Suo*), 元胡索 (*Yuan Hu Suo*), or simply 元胡 (*Yuan Hu*). Some medicinals' names are often abbreviated or contracted. For instance, Rhizoma Imperatae Cylindricae (*Bai Mao Gen*) is often just *Mao Gen*. Flos Lonicerae Japonicae (*Jin Yin Hua*) is often just *Yin Hua*. However, sometimes it is known by its alternative names, 双花 (*Shuang Hua*) or 儿花 (*Er Hua*). Tuber Ophiopogonis Japonici (*Mai Men Dong*) is routinely identified as only *Mai Dong*. Fructus Zizyphi Spinosae (*Suan Zao Ren*) is often identified only as *Zao Ren*. Fructus Gardeniae Jasminoidis (*Shan Zhi Zi*) may be abbreviated as either *Shan Zhi* or *Zhi Zi*. And mix-fried Radix Glycyrrhizae (*Zhi Gan Cao*) is often called simply *Zhi Cao*.

There are also some common abbreviations of groups of medicinals. For instance, Radix Rubrus Paeoniae Lactiflorae (*Chi Shao*) and Radix Albus Paeoniae Lactiflorae (*Bai Shao*) are frequently referred to as *Chi Bai Shao*, while uncooked Radix Rehmanniae (*Sheng Di*) and cooked Radix Rehmanniae (*Shu Di*) when used together are often referred to as *Sheng Shu Di*. Red and White Sclerotium Poriae Cocos are referred to as *Chi Bai Fu Ling*. And the 三仙 (*san xian*) or three immortals are Massa Medica Fermentata (*Shen Shu*), Fructus Crataegi (*Shan Zha*), and Semen Germinatus Hordei Vulgaris (*Mai Ya*).

Fail-safe identifications

The single best way to identify Chinese medicinals is by the Chinese characters. But in-putting Chinese characters every time a medicinal is mentioned is time-consuming, even if you own the software, and in translation and publishing, time means money. If you only use Pinyin to identify a Chinese medicinal, there may be questions when the author uses alternative names or abbreviations.[1] If you just use Latin, there can also be differences of nomenclature, as we have seen between Bensky & Gamble and the *Zhong Yao Da Ci Dian* and cloves.

Therefore, I strongly recommend using both the Pinyin and the Latin pharmacological

---

[1] If you are doing a denotative translation and the author uses *Mai Dong* as their identification, then I believe you must also use *Mai Dong* as your Pinyin identification. If you substitute *Mai Men Dong*, then you have lost the transparency the denotative translation seeks to capture.

nomenclature. This doubling up helps insure the proper identification. If the Pinyin is perplexing, hopefully the Latin will clarify the issue. If the Latin looks peculiar, hopefully the Pinyin will be recognizable. I do not recommend using common English names because the English language literature on Chinese medicine is read all over the world. People in Europe have a better chance of working with the Latin than with common English names. Personally, it doesn't make much difference to me if you put the Pinyin first and the Latin in parentheses or the Latin first and the Pinyin in parentheses. But having both makes your identification as fail-safe as possible short of including the Chinese characters.

20
Going Further

This workbook is only meant to help you get started on what hopefully will be a lifelong exploration of the Chinese medical literature. There are several books which can help you study characters and practice translation. These are all books available in the U.S. which include sections of Chinese text interspersed with that text's English translation. The more you can memorize or at least familiarize yourself with the commonly occurring characters, the less characters you will have to look up in your Chinese-English dictionary. The less characters you have to look up, the faster you can translate.

The first book I would like to recommend is my own *Statements of Fact in TCM*. This small book is a collection of short, pithy sentences which are the key statements of fact in Chinese medicine. Each statement appears in simplified Chinese characters, Pinyin romanization, and English translation using Nigel Wiseman's terminology from 1990. One of the ways I got to be a world famous practitioner and teacher of Chinese medicine is by drilling myself in these statements of fact. The more you look at these statements of fact, both in the English words and Chinese characters, the more you will A) become familiar with the main medical characters and B) familiar with Chinese sentence structure. While the 1994 edition has some typos and I would like to retranslate some of these sentences, it is still a very useful and inexpensive companion piece to this workbook.

Exercise: On page 198 you'll find a sample page reproduced from *Statements of Fact in TCM*. See if you can find the Chinese typos and improve some of the translations in this book. Since the Pinyin is there, looking the characters up in your Pinyin Chinese-English dictionary and in Nigel's dictionary is a snap.

Secondly, I would like to recommend Paul Unschuld's two volume *Learn to Read Chinese* published by Paradigm Publications. This set was created for teaching Unschuld's sinology and medical anthropology students how to read modern medical Chinese. As I have mentioned previously, by itself, I do not think it is a good place for Western Chinese medical students to begin. He has picked a text-dense Chinese text to work with whose content is more theoretical than clinical. However, when supplemented by this workbook, *Learn to Read Chinese* can be very helpful.

Volume 1 of *Learn to Read Chinese* is comprised of excerpts from an introduction to Chinese medicine written by Qin Bo-wei, one of the architects of modern Chinese medicine. These excerpts are first given in Chinese characters and then in Pinyin romanization. Following this, there is a list of new vocabulary, and following that list there is Unschuld's translation. The first part of Vol. 2 analyzes each of the sentences in volume one, diagramming their grammar. This is very helpful for learning how to interpret Chinese sentence structure. The second part of Vol. 2 is an alphabetized index or glossary of all the words in the Chinese source text.

Life Principles

The essence generates the qi (and) the qi generates the spirit.

(*Jing sheng qi, qi sheng shen.* 精生气，气生神)

The kidneys rule water.

(*Shen zhu shui.* 肾主水)

The kidneys are the water viscus; they govern fluids and humor.

(*Shen wei shui zang, zhu jin ye.* 肾为水脏，主津液)

The kidneys govern qi absorption.

(*Shen zhu na qi.* 肾主纳气)

The kidneys govern the bones.

(*shen zhu gu.* 肾主骨)

The bones generate marrow; the brain is the sea of marrow.

(*Gu sheng sui, nao wei sui hai.* 骨生髓，脑为髓海)

The teeth are the surplus of the bones.

(*Chi wei gu zhi yu.* 齿为骨之余)

The cheeks are the roots of the bones.

(*Quan wei gu zhi ben.* 颧为骨之本)

The kidneys are in charge of the two excretions.

(*Shen si er bian.* 肾司二便)

The kidneys control the fire of the gate of life.

(*Shen zhu ming men zhi huo.* 肾主命门之火)

49

Unfortunately, Unschuld does not use Wiseman's terminology. So his rendition is not the same as I have been promoting. Nevertheless, this is an excellent set of books as long as they are not the sole books used to try to learn how to read Chinese. Their format and design is very similar to foreign language texts used for teaching Spanish, French, German, etc. We must remember than Unschuld is teaching postgraduate academics whose sole or at least focus is on their schoolwork. We, on the other hand, are busy adults with families and jobs. If we are in school, it is mostly night school or on weekends. In addition, we are not learning Chinese medicine as scholars but as practitioners. Therefore, my experience as both a student and a teacher is that we need a radically different approach.

The third source to help you in your study and practice of reading modern medical Chinese is Shuai Xue-zhong's *Chinese-English Terminology of Traditional Chinese Medicine* published by the Hunan Science & Technology Press, Changsha, 1983. This book contains compound terms and statements of fact in simplified Chinese characters, Pinyin romanization, and English translation. In some ways, it is similar to my own *Statements of Fact*. However, it is a glossary of single and compound terms as well. It contains chapters on:

1. Yin & Yang and the Five Elements
2. Visceral Symptoms
3. Channels & Their Collateral Channels and Acupuncture Points
4. Etiology & Pathology
5. Techniques of Diagnosis
6. The General Rules of Treatment
7. The Chinese Medical Formulary
8. Acupuncture and Moxibustion
9. Internal Medicine and Pediatrics
10. Gynecology and Obstetrics
11. Surgery and Traumatology
12. The Five Sensory Organs
13. The History of Traditional Chinese Medicine

If you have read the above list of chapter titles carefully, you already know that this book's English translation is at variance from the norms that I am suggesting. In actual fact, I do not think the English translation is very good. However, because there are the simplified characters, the Pinyin, and at least some English translations, this book is a very good one to go through trying to retranslate the English. If you do this, as I have done, you will learn more about Chinese medicine *as Chinese speak about and understand it*, you will begin to see that we cannot rely on native Chinese-speakers for our translations, and you will help familiarize yourself with the main medical characters.

And finally, the fourth book, or actually set of books, I recommend to help you go further is *A Practical English-Chinese Library of Traditional Chinese Medicine* published by the Shanghai College of Traditional Chinese Medicine in Shanghai in 1994. This is a 12 volume set. On the right side of the page is the Chinese text in simplified characters, while on the left side is the English translation. The titles of the volumes in this series are:

Basic Theory of Traditional Chinese Medicine (I)
Basic theory of Traditional Chinese Medicine (II)
Diagnostics of Traditional Chinese Medicine
The Chinese Materia Medica
Prescriptions of Traditional Chinese Medicine
Clinic of Traditional Chinese Medicine (I)
Clinic of Traditional Chinese Medicine (II)
Health Preservation and Rehabilitation
Chinese Acupuncture and Moxibustion
Chinese Massage
Chinese Medicated Diet
Chinese Qigong

The Pinyin of the text is not given in any of these volumes, and, as you will see in the next chapter, I take exception to the quality of the English translation. However, these books are readily available in North America. They can provide you with a very nice, very concise Chinese language library on all the main aspects of Chinese medicine. You can learn a huge amount both about Chinese medicine and translating Chinese medicine if you spend some time comparing what the Chinese says using Nigel Wiseman's terminology and translating denotatively with how the Chinese translators have glossed or paraphrased the text. I believe that once you see for yourself what the Chinese actually says and how the typical native Chinese-speaker fails to capture the technical precision of the original, you will never again be able to complacently read such a Chinese-done translation.

My experience is that, by working with this workbook and the above four other supplementary titles (or sets), you can revolutionize your understanding and clinical practice of Chinese medicine. Try it.

20
Conclusion

Following this last chapter, there are several appendices and an annotated bibliography (called Resources & References) to help you even more in translating modern medical Chinese into English. Appendix 1 is a Pinyin/Wade-Giles/Yale conversion chart. Appendix 2 is a collection of more readings which you can work on as you wait for your first Chinese books and journals to arrive. And Appendix 3 is comprised of more blanks for practicing how to write Chinese characters.

I know that some Chinese reading the following paragraphs are going to accuse me of racism. However, such charges would exemplify the lack of exactly the degree of English proficiency necessary to act as professional Chinese-English translators. I believe that only native English-speakers (be they white, red, yellow, black, brown, or beige) can credibly translate the Chinese medical literature into English. Till now, we have assumed that Chinese people can translate the Chinese medical literature for us into English, that Chinese is a difficult language which somehow we Westerners cannot master. However, I believe that, in professional translation, the translator should be a native speaker of the *arrival* language (in this case English), *not* the departure language (in this case Chinese). It is my many years experience that only native English-speakers have the feel for the English language and understand the Western standards of translation necessary to professionally translate this literature into English.

I say this making my living as a writer, editor, and translator. As of this writing, I have edited almost 30 books on all aspects of Chinese medicine translated originally by native Chinese-speakers. When I have compared these English translations to their Chinese original source texts, what I have found *in every case* was more a functional or at best a connotative translation than a denotative one. In other words, in every case, I have had to retranslate all these texts, word by word, sentence by sentence, paragraph by paragraph until A) they sounded close to a native English-speaker's and B) were faithful to the Chinese original. Now at Blue Poppy Press, we won't even accept translations done by native Chinese-speaking translators unless we have the time and are willing to undertake the complete retranslation of the work.

Below I would like to give a couple of examples of what I find wrong with English language translations done by Chinese. They are both from published sources where the Chinese and English texts are printed side by side. Remember, we are dealing with *Fachprosa,* and a *Fachprosa* which has consequences for the health and even lives of our real-life patients. Therefore, I believe that the technical accuracy and faithfulness required in this endeavor are higher than *any Chinese translator's* I have seen in my 15 years experience as an editor. Although I can read Chinese, I would never in a million years think to write something for publication in Chinese. As anyone who has ever tried to learn a foreign language knows, it is one thing to read and understand a foreign language. It is altogether something else to speak or write in that foreign language. *And English is the hardest language in the world*!

A Coloured Atlas of the Chinese Materia Medica Specified in Pharmacopoeia of the People's Republic of China (1995 Edition) is a handsome and expensive book on Chinese materia medica created in the People's Republic of China but printed in Hong Kong.[1] For each medicinal included there is a Chinese passage (unfortunately written in complicated characters) which is then abbreviated and translated into English. If we look on page 34 under *Shan Zha* (Fructus Crataegi), we will find the following:

034 山楂

Shanzha

Hawthorn Fruit

FRUCTUS CRATAEGI

本品為薔薇科植物山裏紅 Crataegus pinnatifida Bge. var. major N. E. Br. 或山楂 Crataegus pinnatifida Bge. 的乾燥成熟果實。

〔原植物〕①山裏紅：落葉小喬木，高約 6m．無刺或疏生短刺。葉互生，具托葉．葉片菱狀卵形，具5～9羽狀淺裂．邊緣有不規則重鋸齒。傘房花序．花白色或稍帶紅暈。梨果球形，直徑達 2.5cm．深亮紅色。②山楂：葉3～5羽狀淺裂。果實直徑 1～1.5cm，深紅色。

〔藥材性狀〕本品為圓形片，皺縮不平．直徑 1～2.5cm．厚 0.2～0.4cm。外皮紅色．具皺紋．有灰白小斑點。果肉深黃色至淺棕色。中部橫切片具5粒淺黃色果核．但核多脫落而中空。有的片上可見短而細的果梗或花萼殘迹。

〔性味功能與主治〕酸、甘、微溫。消食健胃．行氣散瘀。用於肉食積滯．胃脘脹滿．瀉痢腹痛．瘀血經閉．產後瘀阻．心腹刺痛．疝氣疼痛；高血脂症。焦山楂消食導滯作用增強。用於肉食積滯．瀉痢不爽。

〔用法與用量〕9～12g。

Hawthorn Fruit is the dried dripe fruit of *Crataegus pinnatifida* Bge. var *major* N. E. Br. or *Crataegus pinnatifida* Bge. (Fam. Rosaceae).

Action To stimulate digestion and promote the functional activity of the stomach. to improve the normal flow of *qi* and dissipate *blood stasis*.

Indications Stagnation of undigested meat with epigastric distension. diarrhea and abdominal pain; amenorrhea due to *blood stasis*. epigastric pain or abdominal colic. after childbirth; heraial pain; hyperlipemia.

Fructus Crataegi (charred): Has more digestant action and is particularly useful for stagnation of undigested meat and diarrhea with inadequate discharge from the bowels.

Dosage 9～12g.

---

[1] Pharmacopoeia Commission of the Ministry of Public Health, P.R. China, *A Coloured Atlas of the Chinese Materia Medica Specified in Pharmacopoeia of the People's Republic of China*, Joint Publishing (H.K.), Co., Ltd. Hong Kong, 1996

In Chinese, the bold-faced heading says: Nature, flavor(s), functions, and indications. This is followed by:

> Sour, sweet, and slightly warm. Disperses food and fortifies the stomach, moves the qi and scatters stasis. It is used for meat food accumulation and stagnation, stomach venter distention and fullness, diarrhea and dysentery abdominal pain, static blood menstrual block, postpartum stasis obstruction, heart and abdominal piercing pain, mounting qi aching and pain, and hyperlipidemia. Scorched Fructus Crataegi's effect of dispersing food and abducting stagnation is even stronger. It is used for meat food accumulation and stagnation, diarrhea and dysentery not straightforward (*i.e.*, incompletely discharged). [Parentheses mine]

In English, this same section is "translated" thus:

> **Action** To stimulate digestion and promote the functional activity of the stomach, to improve the normal flow of *qi* and dissipate *blood stasis*.

> **Indications** Stagnation of undigested meat with epigastric distention, diarrhea and abdominal pain; amenorrhea due to *blood stasis*, epigastric pain or abdominal colic, after childbirth; heraial [*sic*] pain; hyperlipidemia.

> *Fructus Crataegi (charred)*: Has more digestant action and is particularly useful for stagnation of undigested meat and diarrhea with inadequate discharge from the bowels.

If you compare these two sections you will notice that the heading is not completely translated and is broken up into two divisions not in keeping with the Chinese source text. There is no mention of the nature and flavors in either the heading or the following text. Then the rest of the text is functionally translated or glossed without retaining the technical vocabulary necessary for a practitioner's understanding and use. Stimulating the digestion and promoting the functional activity of the stomach, improving the normal flow of the qi and dissipating blood stasis may be ultimately what this passage means in a non-technical format, but that is very different from what the text actually says if one renders it verbatim using Nigel Wiseman's terminology. This is, in my experience, par for the course for a translation from Chinese to English concerning the practice of Chinese medicine done by a native Chinese-speaker. However, so you will not think this is an isolated case, let's look at another example.

The following section comes from *A Practical English-Chinese Library of Traditional Chinese Medicine: The Chinese Materia Medica* published by the Shanghai College of Traditional Chinese Medicine Publishing House.[2] This is a 12 volume series on Chinese medicine created by a school with a long history of teaching the clinical practice of Chinese medicine to foreigners in English. This section is on *Chuan Shan Jia* (Squama Mantidis Pentadactylis, 穿山甲).

---

[2] *A Practical English-Chinese Library of Traditional Chinese Medicine: The Chinese Materia Medica*, ed. by Zhang En-qin, Shanghai College of Traditional Chinese Medicine, Shanghai, 1990, p. 312-313

穿 山 甲

为鲮鲤科动物食蚁鲮鲤的鳞片。产于广西、贵州、广东、云南、台湾等地。捕后杀死，割下整张甲壳，置沸水中烫过，取下鳞片，洗净晒干，与砂同炒至松脆起泡而呈黄色后用；或炒后趁热置醋内略浸，晒干备用。

【性味归经】 咸，微寒。归肝、胃经。

【功效】 活血通经，下乳，消肿排脓。

【应用】

1. 用于血滞经闭、癥瘕积块，以及风湿痹痛等。如治经闭，可配当归、川芎、牛膝、红花；治癥瘕，可配三棱、莪术；治痹痛，可配羌活、防风、苏木等。

2. 用于乳汁不通。常与王不留行配伍。若兼肝郁乳胀者，可配柴胡、青皮；因产后气血不足而乳汁稀少者，须与黄芪、当归等同用。

3. 用于疮痈肿痛。若初起尚未成脓者，常与金银花、天花粉、赤芍等配伍，如仙方活命饮；脓成未溃者，常与皂角刺、当归、黄芪等同用，如透脓散。

【用量用法】 3～10克，水煎服。亦可研末吞服，每次1～1.5克。以研末吞服效果较好。

【使用注意】 孕妇及痈疽已溃者忌用。

The English translation on page 312 begins well enough. It says, "This drug is the scales of *Mantis pentadactyla L.* (Family *Mandae*) which is produced in *Guangxi, Guizhou, Guangdong, Yunnan* and *Taiwan* provinces." In Chinese, there are two sentences here separated by a period, but this is no big deal. Then it goes on to say, "The killed pangolin is skinned to get the whole skin with scales which is put into boiling water to be scaled off the scales." This is not very good English, but I still don't have a real problem with this translation. It simply wasn't edited well. It goes on to say, "The scales are collected and washed clean, dried in sunlight, stir-baked with sand till the scales are light and crisp, bulgy, and yellow in colour, or stir-baked and then, while hot, soaked in vinegar for a short period, and dried for use." In this sentence we have some problems which actually have practical, real-life consequences. First of all, baking means baking in an oven. There is no such processing form in Chinese medicine as "stir-baking". The term is stir-frying. This implies frying in a wok on top of a stove or open flame. The text goes on to say that these are stir-fried until light and crisp (the meaning of 松 *song* and 脆 *cui*) and they become "bulgy." There is no such word in English and this adjective is meaningless as a description of the goal of this processing method. The Chinese is 起 (*qi*), to rise, 泡 (*pao*), like a bubble. If you have seen this processing method done, the scales puff up like dough rising or popcorn puffing up. To bulge means "to become lumpy". Here the meaning is "to puff up". This particular verb should have been handled with a footnote explaining what to rise like a bubble means in this context. The rest of the sentence is ok.

The bold-faced, bracketed heading which comes next, says, "Nature, flavor(s), and channel gathering(s)." It is rendered by the Chinese translator as, "Property, flavour and channel tropism." The translation goes on to say, "Salty in flavour, slightly cold in property, acting on the liver and stomach channels." Why the translator has used two different words to translate (*Gui*) is not clear. In both instances, the meaning is the same. This verb is definitely not the verb "to act on". However, at least the translator did translate this section, unlike the translator of the section from the other book above.

The next bold-faced, bracketed heading says, "Effects." I'm ok with that. "Clearing away obstruction in the channels by promoting blood circulation, stimulating milk secretion, subduing swelling, and promoting the drainage of pus" is, however, not only grammatically incorrect, it is far from the technical meaning of these terms. I would translate this passage thus: "Quickens the blood and frees the flow of the channels, descends (or precipitates) the milk, disperses swelling and expels pus."

Then we come to the bold-faced, bracketed heading 应用 (*Ying yong*), "Indications." Ok, we can go with that. The first indication is rendered: "1. Amenorrhea and masses in the abdomen due to stagnation of blood, and rheumatic arthralgia..." I would render this line as, "Used for blood stagnation menstrual block, concretions and conglomerations, accumulations and lumps as well as wind damp impediment pain." While *jing bi* can be translated as "amenorrhea" when it appears in a Western medical context, I believe it should be translated as "menstrual block", literally what the words say, when this term is used in a Chinese medical context. Amenorrhea is Greek for no monthly or menstrual flow. In the Chinese medical literature, blocked menstruation is defined as being different from the normal absence of menstruation. Rather it is a pathological condition and one of the traditional disease categories listed under menstrual diseases (月径病，

yue jing bing) in Chinese gynecology (妇科, *fu ke*). As such, it is the yin-yang opposite of *beng lou* (迸, flooding, and 漏, leaking). The character for block in menstrual block shows a door sealed shut, while the characters for *beng lou* both imply something erroneously open and letting something which should be dammed up flow out.

The second indication is rendered: "2. Galactostasis" Huh? As I read it, it says quite plainly, "Used for breast milk which is not freely flowing." There is no word "galactostasis" in my copy of *The Merck Manual* or *The New American Medical Dictionary and Health Manual*. And stasis and lack of free flow are two different concepts. Although they often go together, they are *not* identical.

The third indication is rendered: "3. Sores, carbuncles, and other pyogenic skin infections." As I read it, it says, "Used for sores and welling abscesses, swelling and pain." I see no mention of other, pyogenic skin infections.

The clinical practice of Chinese medicine is based, in large degree, on the precise use of certain technical terms which then lead to the precise selection of appropriate remedies. If you gloss over the technical lingo, you loose the precision of the medicine.

Jürgen Kovacs, in his article, "Linguistic Reflections on the Translation of Chinese Medical Texts", makes the same observation on the limitation of Chinese translators which I have experienced since 1983: "For those who translate from their own language into a foreign language, *e.g.*, from... Chinese into English, it can be proven by countless examples that their approach to the source language text is too strongly influenced by intuition and that their rendering in English appears unbalanced by the failure to choose and maintain the correct stylistic, communicative, and connotative level."[3]

I first became involved with the technical issues surrounding translation when helping to translate a Buddhist text from Tibetan to English in the early 1970s. In ancient Tibet, translations from Sanskrit to Tibetan were often done by committees. In that case, the ideal committee was made up of the following experts (some of which might actually be the same person):

1) A native Sanskrit-speaking expert in the technical subject about which the Sanskrit text was written

2) A native Sanskrit-speaking scholar of the Sanskrit language

3) A native Sanskrit-speaking Sanskrit-Tibetan translator

4) A native Tibetan-speaking Sanskrit-Tibetan translator

5) A native Tibetan-speaking scholar of the Tibetan language

---

[3] Kovacs, Jürgen, *op. cit.*, p. 94

206

6) A native Tibetan-speaking expert in the technical subject

In other words, there are at least six different types of expertise necessary to do a faithful, denotative, technical translation, and a committee made up of all six of these areas of expertise is probably the best way to insure a high degree of accuracy *and* fluency in a *Fachprosa* translation. These Sanskrit-Tibetan translators were not satisfied unless some other translators could put the Tibetan work back into Sanskrit with a high degree of accuracy. Doing denotative translation with a standard technical vocabulary, you can also do this with English translations of modern Chinese medical literature.

In fact, the Blue Poppy Press books in our Great Masters Series are done by such a committee. Yang Shou-zhong is 1) a classical Chinese scholar, 2) a practitioner of Chinese medicine, and 3) a professor of English at the college level. When he has questions about the Chinese medical content of a translation he is working on and he cannot find the answer in some book, he goes to various professors at the TCM college he teaches at or writes to TCM authorities around the PRC. Likewise, when faced with a question about classical Chinese grammar or usage, Mr. Yang seeks out the advice and in-put of Chinese linguistic scholars. In addition, although only Mr. Yang's name typically appears as translator of this series, I go over every line. I have 4) been writing English professionally since I was 15, 5) have been a practitioner of Chinese medicine for 20 years, and 6) have translated a number of Chinese books and scores of articles into English on my own. If I have questions about the technical medical meaning of a Chinese word or phrase, I often ask a local native Chinese-speaking Chinese doctor, such as Zhang Ting-liang, Gao Yu-li, or Zhou Ming-ying. Or I may ask questions of other native English-speaking Chinese medical translators who regularly work with Blue Poppy, such as Charles (Chip) Chace and Lance Halvorsen, or one of the professors in the Chinese department at Colorado University. Therefore, our team does encompass the various skills enumerated above. After I edit Mr. Yang's version, it gets sent back to Mr. Yang for him to approve my changes. Only when we both agree is one of our books ready for publication.

In any case, I believe it is imperative that we English-speaking practitioners of Chinese medicine wake up to the fact that the onus of translating the Chinese medical literature into English rests squarely on us. We must not abrogate this responsibility out of either laziness or ignorance. Native Chinese-speakers *by themselves* do not have the English language skills to discharge this role. And native English-speakers who are not A) Chinese medical practitioners themselves and B) highly educated authorities on the English language are not much help.[4]

For sure, we native English-speakers must frequently and with humility turn to our native Chinese-speaking peers to ask for their advice, their interpretation, their understanding of difficult words and passages, and, as mentioned above, I believe it is best when a translation is done as a joint affair between native Chinese and native English speakers. However, I strongly believe it is we native English-speaking professional practitioners of Chinese medicine who must

---

[4] I mention this fact because often, so-called foreign experts working in China are listed as the editors or consultants on English language Chinese medical projects. In my experience, such helpers have never possessed what I consider to be the necessary qualifications for such a job. Just being a native speaker is not enough. You can be a good, skilled, and knowledgable native speaker or a poor, unskilled, and linguistically uneducated native speaker.

create and constantly enlarge the English language literature of this profession translated from Chinese. If this workbook helps even one more person begin translating the Chinese medical literature into English, the time and effort I have put into creating it will have been worth it. To me, our very survival as an mature, reliable, independent health care profession depends, at least in part, on our shouldering of this burden.

Closing words

I know you can teach yourself how to read modern medical Chinese. I know this because I myself have done it. I am not saying that this is an easy task. It is time-consuming, sometimes boring, and sometimes frustrating. But I feel very strongly that the time and effort are well worth it. In the chapters above, I have given you a number of hints on how to approach this piece of work. Now it's up to you to follow through and practice. When the great Tibetan yogi, Milarepa, was saying good-bye to his foremost student, Gampopa, he wanted to give this student a last, most important piece of advice. So Milarepa lifted his skirt and showed Gampopa his butt which was callused by decades of sitting *practicing* meditation.

As I write this conclusion, my current *Pinyin Chinese-English Dictionary* is falling to pieces in my hands. If you don't have to buy a new Chinese-English dictionary every year or so, you're not practicing translating enough. If you use your Chinese-English dictionary, you will literally wear it out. Then you know you are persevering. If you're not persevering, no one can pour the ability to translate modern medical Chinese into your mind while watching TV.

If you do persevere and do succeed in creating one or more denotative translations, don't forget to keep Blue Poppy Press in mind as a publisher. If you spend the time to translate something from Chinese, then I believe it is your ethical obligation to share that knowledge with our entire profession. Although there are many dozens more books on Chinese medicine now than when I started out as a student in 1976-77, there are still too few books to really credibly train doctoral level practitioners. Until that literature is available to anyone wanting to become a doctor of Chinese medicine, I believe we each must contribute all that we can.

Good luck.

Resources & References

Chinese-English Dictionaries

The Pinyin Chinese-English Dictionary, ed. by Wu Jing-rong, Beijing Foreign Languages Institute, The Commercial Press , Beijing & Hong Kong, and John Wiley and Sons, Inc. New York, 1991, available in both hard and soft-backed editions. This is the recommended basic Chinese-English dictionary. Although the print is a little small, it is paperbound and can be flipped through easily.

The Chinese-English Dictionary, Heian International Press, Union City, CA. This is very similar to the above dictionary and, in fact, was originally published by The Commercial Press, Hong Kong, 1979. However, it contains less characters. It is also a paperback. It will do to get you started if it is all you can find, but, for the same money, buy the first one if you can.

A Chinese-English Dictionary, ed. by Wu Jin-rong, Beijing Foreign Languages Institute, the Commercial Press, Beijing, 1988. The text of this book is identical to the first dictionary listed above. However, the print is larger. This makes it easier for beginner's to decipher the characters. On the other hand, it is hard bound; so you cannot flip through it, and the quality of the paper is poor and tends to rip easily.

Mathew's Chinese-English Dictionary, R.H. Mathews, Harvard University Press, Cambridge, MA, 1979. This dictionary is for looking up so-called complicated characters. It is also useful for looking up characters whose radicals are obscure. It uses the Wade-Giles system of romanization. You can convert this into Pinyin by using Appendix 1 below.

A Reverse Chinese-English Dictionary, Yu Yun-xia *et al.*, The Commercial Press, Beijing, 1985. This dictionary is useful if you cannot find the first word of a two character compound term. In that case, you first look up the second character in your Pinyin Chinese-English dictionary. Then, armed with the Pinyin spelling, you look up this character in this "reverse" Chinese-English dictionary. Next, scan the list of compounds for the first character. Once found, it does give the Pinyin, although it still doesn't help you to look up the character in question from scratch.

Chinese-English Medical Dictionary, ed. by Cui Yue-li, The Commercial Press/People's Health & Hygiene Press, Beijing & Hong Kong, 1988. This is the best Chinese-English medical dictionary I have seen. Although it includes some Chinese medicine, the emphasis is overwhelmingly on modern Western medicine. This book is indispensable when trying to translate journal articles which tend to start with Western medical diseases and typically include Western medical information.

Chinese-English Terminology of Traditional Chinese Medicine, Shuai Xue-zhong, Hunan Science & Technology Press, Changsha, 1983. Although the translations are only connotative, this is a good listing of most of the important terms and statements of fact of Chinese medicine.

Han Ying Chong Yong Yi Xue Ci Hui (A Collection of Commonly Used Chinese-English Medical Words), People's Health & Hygiene Press, Beijing, 1982. This is also a Chinese-English medical dictionary. It contains somewhat different vocabulary from the first Chinese-English medical dictionary listed above. It includes both Western and Chinese medical terms, with the emphasis on the Western medicine.

Chinese English Dictionary of Function Words, ed. by Wang Hai, Sinolingua, Beijing, 1992. This book is devoted to grammatical and other such function words. These words are often not defined in the *Pinyin Chinese-English Dictionary.* In many cases, that dictionary only gives examples of how the word is used in a Chinese sentence. This book also primarily gives examples, but does also supply succinct definitions and English language explanations. I have included many of these words in the general or linking word list in chapter 14 above.

English-Chinese Dictionaries

Practical Dictionary of Chinese Medicine, Nigel Wiseman & Feng Ye, Paradigm Publications, Brookline, MA 1998. This is, quite simply, one of the most important and valuable books about Chinese medicine in English. In it, Wiseman and Feng give definitions of all their term suggestions. These definitions help clarify the technical nuances of those terms. No translator of Chinese medicine can afford to be without this book.

A New English-Chinese Dictionary, The Commercial Press, Beijing & Hong Kong, 1985. This dictionary can be useful if you cannot find a character but you think you know what it means in English. In that case, look up the word in English and see if the character in question is given as a possible Chinese translation or equivalent.

English-Chinese Medical Dictionary, The Commercial Press/People's Health & Hygiene Press, Beijing & Hong Kong, 1995. This dictionary is the reverse of the *Chinese-English Medical Dictionary* mentioned above in the preceding section. If you are having trouble finding the translation of what you think are Western medical terms and you think you might know what those terms are, then you can look them up in English in this dictionary and see if you are correct. This dictionary is also very useful for determining the Chinese characters for diseases you may be interested in. Armed with a knowledge of the characters for emphysema or cervical neoplasia, you can then keep your eyes open for these when scanning the tables of contents of books and journals.

Western Names for Chinese Disease Classes, Hong-yen Hsu, Oriental Healing Arts Institute, Long Beach, CA, 1990. Although this book is not very big and the Chinese characters are written in their traditional, complicated forms, this book is a nice little listing of Western disease names and their Chinese equivalents. Because this book was compiled by a Taiwanese author, in many cases, it gives slightly different names than those found in the above medical dictionaries from the PRC. This allows for a broader search when both these resources are used together.

Chinese-Chinese Dictionaries

At first, the idea of using a Chinese-Chinese dictionary may be daunting. However, as your ability to read Chinese improves, you will undoubtedly run across words, book titles, names, and medicinals which you cannot find in your various Chinese-English dictionaries and glossaries. In this case, you will need to go to various Chinese-Chinese dictionaries and encyclopedia. Below are the one's I find I use fairly regularly.

中药大词典 *(Zhong Yao Da Ci Dian, Dictionary of Chinese Medicinals)*, Zhejiang College of New Medicine, Shanghai Science & Technology Press, Shanghai 1986. This is a standard materia medica reference text with more than 5,700 medicinals. It is the single best source of information on Chinese medicinals I know of in any language.

简明中医词典 *(Jian Ming Zhong Yi Ci Dian, Simple & Clear Chinese Medicine Dictionary)*, People's Health & Hygiene Press, Beijing, 1979. This is a good dictionary for looking up Chinese medical terms, medicinals, formulas, authors, etc.

针灸学词典 *(Zhen Jiu Xue Ci Dian, A Dictionary of Acupuncture & Moxibustion)*, Anhui College of Chinese Medicine & Shanghai College of Chinese Medicine, Shanghai Science & Technology Press, Shanghai, 1987. This is a good dictionary for looking up terms related to specifically to acupuncture and moxibustion, especially unusual acupuncture points.

中医人名词典 *(Zhong Yi Ren Ming Ci Dian, A Dictionary of Chinese Medical Personages' Names)*, Li Yun, International Culture Publishing Company, Beijing, 1988. This book can help you identify Chinese medical personages mentioned in other Chinese language sources. It tells where they were born, when they lived, what they wrote, their style names, and other important points in terms of their fame as Chinese doctors .

中药别名手册 *(Zhong Yao Bie Ming Shou Ce, A Handbook of Chinese Medicinal Alternative Names)*, Bao Xi-sheng, Guangdong Science & Technology Press, Guangzhou, 1993. This book is very useful for identifying Chinese medicinals when authors use alternative names.

中医古籍珍本提要 *(Zhong Yi Gu Ji Zhen Ben Ti Yao, A Synopsis of Chinese Medicine Ancient Records & Rare Books)*, Yu Ying-ao & Fu Jing-hua, Chinese Medicine Ancient Books Press, Beijing, 1992. This book is a handy reference for identifying books mentioned in passing in other Chinese sources. It identifies the book's author, date of publication, contents, and why it is important in the history of Chinese medicine .

Standard Glossaries

Glossary of Chinese Medical Terms and Acupuncture Points, Nigel Wiseman, Paradigm Publications, Brookline, MA, 1990. This is Nigel's first published Chinese-English English-Chinese Chinese medical glossary. It has been supplanted by the following title. However, if you cannot find the following title, this glossary is still ok to begin with. Most of the terms are the same. It also includes a very good essay on the importance of adopting a standard translational terminology based on a freely available glossary.

English-Chinese Chinese-English Dictionary of Chinese Medicine, Nigel Wiseman, Hunan Science & Technology Press, Changsha, 1995. This is Nigel's updated, revised glossary. In it, all updated terms have been marked, giving both Nigel's original term and his revised term. In addition, this glossary includes Chinese medicinals and formulas which the 1990 Paradigm version does not. However, please note, this is not a dictionary since it does not include definitions. It really is a glossary.

English-English References on Chinese & Western Medicine

Descriptions of the usefulness and special features of each of the first five books listed below are given in chapter 18 above.

Chinese Herbal Medicine: Materia Medica, Dan Bensky & Andrew Gamble, Eastland Press, Seattle, 1993

Chinese Herbal Medicine: Formulas & Strategies, Dan Bensky & Randall Barolet, Eastland Press, Seattle, 1990

Oriental Materia Medica: A Concise Guide, Hong-yen Hsu *et al.*, Oriental Healing Arts Institute, Long Beach, CA, 1986

Chinese Materia Medica, Vol. 1-6, Southern Materials Center, Inc., Taipei, 1979

A Barefoot Doctor's Manual, Revolutionary Health Committee of Hunan Province, Cloudburst Press, Mayne Isle & Seattle, 1977

Acupuncture: A Comprehensive Text, trans. & ed. by John O'Connor & Dan Bensky, Eastland Press, Seattle, 1981. This is a very good basic acupuncture text that, unfortunately, has never gotten the attention it deserves. It's a little hard to look points up in this book, since they are not discussed according to the flow of the channels but rather by body parts. Personally, I think the extra channel extraordinary point index and the way these extra points are notated is very good.

The Merck Manual, ed. by Robert Berkow, Merck Sharp & Dohme Research Laboratories, Rahway, NJ, please see whatever is the latest edition. This book is the clinical "bible" of Western medicine. It is basic primer on the definition, etiology, symptomology, diagnosis, and treatment of disease with modern Western medicine. A new edition is published every three or four years.

More Books on Learning Chinese

Chinese Character Exercise Book, Sinolingua, Beijing, 1987. This book contains numerous practice sheets and instructions for learning to write Chinese characters correctly.

Learn to Write Chinese Characters, Johan Björkstén, Yale University Press, New Haven & London, 1994. This is a nicely done little book about different styles of calligraphy and how to write *kai shu.*

Read and Write Chinese: A Simplified Guide to the Chinese Characters, Rita Mei-wah Choy, China West Books, San Francisco, 1990. This book shows the stroke order for hundreds of Chinese characters. The characters included in this book are the complicated or traditional characters. Of particular interest, the author has identified the 300 most frequently used characters that make up 65% of printed materials, 700 more which bring that percentage up to 88%, and 2,210 additional characters which then account for 99% of printed materials. However, keep in mind that the author is talking about reading a newspaper or magazine, not a book or journal specializing in Chinese medicine.

Reading & Writing Chinese by William McNaughton, Charles E. Tuttle Company, Inc. Rutland, VT, 1996. This book presents the correct way to write and the etymological derivation of the 1,020 most useful characters for students of general Chinese according to a consensus of American Chinese language teachers. In addition, it contains the official list of 2,000 characters published in the PRC for adult education. Although many of the characters are the old, "complex" characters, this is a very useful book.

Understanding Chinese Characters by their Ancestral Forms by Ping-gam Go, Simplex Publications, SF, 1995. This is a very easy book designed for novices getting started recognizing and deciphering Chinese characters. As illustrations, it uses advertising signs in San Francisco's Chinatown. Again, many of the characters are the complex or "long form" ones. However, this is a very useful, fun book. It also gives the etymology and evolution of a number of important characters.

I Can Read That: A Traveler's Introduction to Chinese Characters by Julie Mazel Sussman, China Books, SF, 1994. Similar to the above, the author presents a number of basic Chinese characters seen on common signs when traveling in Chinese-speaking countries and areas. Both this and the book above are great ways to demystify written Chinese and both are a lot of fun to go through.

Peng's Chinese Treasury Chinese Radicals, Vol. 1 & 2, by Tan Huay Peng, Heian International, Inc., Torrance, CA, 1987. This two volume set of little books discusses the Chinese radicals under categories, such as radicals having to do with humans, plants, animals, etc. It gives the etymology of the radicals and examples of common characters made from the radicals and illustrates all this with very delightful if slightly kitschy cartoons. This is yet another fun and easy way to learn to recognize and read Chinese.

Beginning Standard Chinese, Helen T. Lin, Sinolingua, Beijing, 1990. This book is a beginning textbook for learning spoken Chinese. However, it includes a lot of useful vocabulary and grammar for those who would like to actually study Chinese grammar.

Teach Yourself Chinese: A Complete Course for Beginners by Elizabeth Scurfield, NTC Publishing Group, Chicago, 1975. Like the above title, this book concentrates on spoken Chinese. However, it is a good source for simple grammar and general vocabulary.

Chinese Characters: Their Origin, Etymology, History, Classification and Signification, L. Weiger, Dover Publications, NY, 1965. This is a reprint of a book which was first published in 1915, so its design and type styles are archaic by contemporary standards. However, this book is a sort of classic in its field, and, just as *Matthew's* is referred to by one name only, most sinologists simply refer to this book as "Weiger." This book gives the etymology or the graphic meaning and development of a host of common Chinese characters. Taken from Chinese sources, these etymologies are the stories Chinese have traditionally told about their characters. Modern research has shown that not all these etymologies are historically accurate. Nevertheless, the make interesting reading and are a helpful way to remember characters. Obviously from the date of the original, this book deals with the complicated or traditional orthography of the characters.

Approaches to Traditional Chinese Medical Literature, ed. by Paul U. Unschuld, Kluwer Academic Publishers, Dordrecht, Boston & London, 1989. This book is a collection of essays about translating Chinese medical texts into English. While some of the essays are a bit esoteric, they nonetheless highlight that the translation of Chinese medicine into English requires special training and skills. Just because one is a native Chinese-speaker does not mean one is qualified to professionally translate medical Chinese, whether classical or modern. Translation, like teaching, is its own profession, and, just because one is an accomplished clinician, does not mean one has the credentials to translate for publication.

About the Chinese language

The Chinese Language: Fact and Fantasy by John De Frnacis. Univ. of Hawaii Press, Honolulu, 1984. This book is a very readable and often humorous technical description of the Chinese language. It dispels many myths about Chinese. It is not necessary to read this book in order to learn how to read Chinese, but if you'd like to understand more about how linguists see Chinese, this is an indispensible book.

Appendix 1:
Pinyin/Wade-Giles/Yale Romanization Conversions

Pinyin is the system of romanization used in the People's Republic of China. It is also the choice of most Chinese-English Chinese medical translators, teachers, and practitioners, at least in the last 15 years since the ascendancy of the TCM style of Chinese medicine. The Wade-Giles system is primarily used these days in Taiwan, Hong Kong, and Singapore. However, it is commonly used in older English language books on Chinese medicine. The Yale system is used by many North American sinologists and medical anthropologists. It does not use the complicated orthography of the Wade-Giles system but is closer to North American norms of pronunciation (as opposed to Pinyin which is based on Russian!).

When hunting down some obscure character or Chinese medicinal, you may have to move from one system of romanization to another. Therefore, the following conversion chart is given in order to make this task a little easier.

Pinyin	Wade-Giles	Yale
a	a	a
ai	ai	ai
an	an	an
ang	ang	ang
ao	ao	au
ba	pa	ba
bai	pai	bai
ban	pan	ban
bang	pang	bang
bao	pao	bao
bei	pei	bei
ben	pên	ben
beng	pêng	beng
bi	pi	bi
bian	pien	byan
biao	piao	byau
bie	pieh	bye
bin	pin	bin
bing	ping	bing
bo	po	bo
bu	pu	bu
ca	ts'a	tsa
cai	ts'ai	tsai
can	ts'an	tsan
cang	ts'ang	tsang
cao	ts'ao	tsau
ce	ts'ê	tse

cen	ts'ên	tsen
ceng	ts'êng	tseng
cha	ch'a	cha
chai	ch'ai	chai
chan	ch'an	chan
chang	ch'ang	chang
chao	ch'ao	chau
che	ch'ê	che
chen	ch'ên	chen
cheng	ch'êng	cheng
chi	ch'ih	chr
chong	ch'ung	chung
chou	ch'ou	chou
chu	ch'u	chu
chua	ch'ua	chwa
chuai	ch'uai	chwai
chuan	ch'uan	chwan
chuang	ch'uang	chwang
chui	ch'ui	chwei
chun	ch'un	chwun
chuo	ch'o	chwo
ci	tz'û	tse
cong	ts'ung	tsung
cou	ts'ou	tsou
cu	ts'u	tsu
cuan	ts'uan	tswan
cui	ts'ui	tswei
cun	ts'un	tswun
cuo	ts'o	tswo
da	ta	da
dai	tai	dai
dan	tan	dan
dang	tang	dang
dao	tao	dau
de	tê	de
deng	têng	deng
di	ti	di
dian	tien	dyan
diao	tiao	dyau
die	tieh	dye
ding	ting	ding
diu	tiu	dyou
dong	tung	dung
dou	tou	dou
du	tu	du
duan	tuan	dwan
dui	tui	dwei
dun	tun	dwun
duo	to	dwo
e	ê	e

ê	eh	
ei	ei	ei
en	ên	en
eng	êng	
er	êrh	er
fa	fa	fa
fan	fan	fan
fang	fang	fang
fei	fei	fei
fen	fên	fen
feng	fêng	feng
fo	fo	fo
fou	fou	fou
fu	fu	fu
ga	ka	ga
gai	kai	gai
gan	kan	gan
gang	kang	gang
gao	kao	gau
ge	kê or ko	ge
gei	kei	gei
gen	kên	gen
geng	kêng	geng
gong	kung	gung
gou	kou	gou
gu	ku	gu
gua	kua	gwa
guai	kuai	gwai
guan	kuan	gwan
guang	kuang	gwang
gui	kui	gwei
gun	kun	gwun
guo	kuo	gwo
ha	ha	ha
hai	hai	hai
han	han	han
hang	hang	hang
hao	hao	hao
he	hê or ho	he
hei	hei	hei
hen	hên	hen
heng	hêng	heng
hong	hung	hung
hou	hou	hou
hu	hu	hu
hua	hua	hwa
huai	huai	hwai
huan	huan	hwan
huang	huang	hwang
hui	hui	hwei

hun	hun	hwun
huo	huo	hwo
ji	chi	ji
jia	chia	jya
jian	chien	jyan
jiang	chiang	jyang
jiao	chiao	jyau
jie	chieh	jye
jin	chin	jin
jing	ching	jing
jiong	chiung	jyung
jiu	chiu	jyou
ju	chü	jyu
juan	chüan	jywan
jue	chüe or chüo	jywe
jun	chün	jyun
ka	k'a	ka
kai	k'ai	kai
kan	k'an	kan
kang	k'ang	kang
kao	k'ao	kau
ke	k'ê or k'o	ke
ken	k'ên	ken
keng	k'êng	keng
kong	k'ung	kung
kou	k'ou	kou
ku	k'u	ku
kua	k'ua	kwa
kuai	k'uai	kwai
kuan	k'uan	kwan
kuang	k'uang	kwang
kui	k'ui	kwei
kun	k'un	kwun
kuo	k'uo	kwo
la	la	la
lai	lai	lai
lan	lan	lan
lang	lang	lang
lao	lao	lau
le	lê or lo	le
lei	lei	lei
leng	lêng	leng
li	li	li
lia	lia	lya
lian	lien	lyan
liang	liang	lyang
liao	liao	lyau
lie	lieh	lye
lin	lin	lin
ling	ling	ling

liu	liu	lyou
long	lung	lung
lou	lou	lou
lu	lu	lu
lü	lü	lyu
luan	luan	lwan
lüe	lüeh, lüo or lio	lywe
lun	lun	lwun
luo	luo	lwo
ma	ma	ma
mai	mai	mai
man	man	man
mang	mang	mang
mao	mao	mau
me	me	me
mei	mei	mei
men	mên	men
meng	mêng	meng
mi	mi	mi
mian	mien	myan
miao	miao	myau
mie	mieh	mye
min	min	min
ming	ming	ming
miu	miu	myou
mo	mo	mo
mou	mou	mou
mu	mu	mu
na	na	na
nai	nai	nai
nan	nan	nan
nang	nang	nang
nao	nao	nau
ne	nê	ne
nei	nei	nei
nen	nên	nen
neng	nêng	neng
ni	ni	ni
nian	nien	nyan
niang	niang	nyang
niao	niao	nyau
nie	nieh	nye
nin	nin	nin
ning	ning	ning
niu	niu	nyou
nong	nung	nung
nou	nou	nou
nu	nu	nu
nü	nü	nyu
nuan	nuan	nwan

nüe	nüeh, nüo or nio	nywe
nuo	no	
o	o	
ou	ou	ou
pa	p'a	pa
pai	p'ai	pai
pan	p'an	pan
pang	p'ang	pang
pao	p'ao	pau
pei	p'ei	pei
pen	p'ên	pen
peng	p'êng	peng
pi	p'i	pi
pian	p'ien	pyan
piao	p'iao	pyau
pie	p'ieh	pye
pin	p'in	pin
ping	p'ing	ping
po	p'o	po
pou	p'ou	pou
pu	p'u	pu
qi	ch'i	chi
qia	ch'ia	chya
qian	ch'ien	chyan
qiang	ch'iang	chyang
qiao	ch'iao	chyau
qie	ch'ieh	chye
qin	ch'in	chin
qing	ch'ing	ching
qiong	ch'iung	chyung
qiu	ch'iu	chyou
qu	ch'ü	chyu
quan	ch'üan	chywan
que	ch'üeh or ch'üo	chywe
qun	ch'ün	chyun
ran	jan	ran
rang	jang	rang
ren	jên	ren
reng	jêng	reng
ri	jih	r
rong	jung	rung
rou	jou	rou
ru	ju	ru
ruan	juan	rwan
rui	jui	rwei
run	jun	rwun
ruo	jo	rwo
sa	sa	sa
sai	sai	sai
san	san	san

sang	sang	sang
sao	sao	sau
se	sê	se
sen	sên	sen
seng	sêng	seng
sha	sha	sha
shai	shai	shai
shan	shan	shan
shang	shang	shang
shao	shao	shau
she	shê	she
shei	shei	shei
shen	shên	shen
sheng	shêng	sheng
shi	shih	shr
shou	shou	shou
shu	shu	shu
shua	shua	shwa
shuai	shuai	shwai
shuan	shuan	shwan
shuang	shuang	shwang
shui	shui	shwei
shun	shun	shwun
shuo	sho	shwo
si	sû, szû or ssû	sz
song	sung	sung
sou	sou	sou
su	su	su
suan	suan	swan
sui	sui	swei
sun	sun	swun
suo	so	swo
ta	t'a	ta
tai	t'ai	tai
tan	t'an	tan
tang	t'ang	tang
tao	t'ao	tau
te	t'ê	te
teng	t'êng	teng
ti	t'i	ti
tian	t'ien	tyan
tiao	t'iao	tyau
tie	t'ieh	tye
ting	t'ing	ting
tong	t'ung	tung
tou	t'ou	tou
tu	t'u	tu
tuan	t'uan	twan
tui	t'ui	twei
tun	t'un	twun

tuo	t'o	two
wa	wa	wa
wai	wai	wai
wan	wan	wan
wang	wang	wang
wei	wei	wei
wen	wên	wen
weng	wêng	weng
wo	wo	wo
wu	wu	wu
xi	hsi	syi
xia	hsia	sya
xian	hsien	syan
xiang	hsiang	syang
xiao	hsiao	syau
xie	hsieh	sye
xin	hsin	syin
xing	hsing	sying
xiong	hsiung	syung
xiu	hsiu	syou
xu	hsü	syu
xuan	hsüan	sywan
xue	hsüeh or hsüo	sywe
xun	hsün	syun
ya	ya	ya
yan	yen	yan
yang	yang	yang
yao	yao	yau
ye	yeh	ye
yi	yi	yi
yin	yin	yin
ying	ying	ying
yo	yo	yo
yong	yung	yung
you	yu	yu
yu	yü	
yuan	yüen	ywan
yue	yüeh	ywe
yun	yün	yun
za	tsa	dza
zai	tsai	dzai
zan	tsan	dzan
zang	tsang	dzang
zao	tsao	dzau
ze	tsê	dze
zei	tsêi	dzei
zen	tsên	dzen
zeng	tsêng	dzeng
zha	cha	ja
zhai	chai	jai

zhan	chan	jan
zhang	chang	jang
zhao	chao	jau
zhe	chê	je
zhei	chei	jei
zhen	chên	jen
zheng	chêng	jeng
zhi	chih	jr
zhong	chung	jung
zhou	chou	jou
zhu	chu	ju
zhua	chua	jwa
zhuai	chuai	jwai
zhuan	chuan	jwan
zhuang	chuang	jwang
zhui	chui	jwei
zhun	chun	jwun
zhuo	cho	jwo
zi	tzû or tsû	dz
zong	tsung	dzung
zou	tsou	dzou
zu	tsu	dzu
zuan	tsuan	dzwan
zui	tsui	dzwei
zun	tsun	dzwun
zuo	tso	dzwo

Appendix 2:
More Texts to Practice On

Zhong Yi Nei Ke Xue (*A Study of Chinese Internal Medicine*) **p. 214-217**
Tetany Condition (includes all types of spasticity and tremors)

36 痉证

痉证是以项背强急, 四肢抽搐, 甚至角弓反张为主要表现的病证。可见于多种疾病。历代医家对痉证的发病原因, 从外感致痉逐步认识到内伤亦可致痉。由于病因学说的丰富和发展, 给痉证治疗不断开创了新的途径。《内经》对痉证的病因是以外邪立论为主, 认为系风寒湿邪, 侵袭人体, 壅阻经络而成。如《素问·至真要大论篇》说: "诸痉项强, 皆属于湿", "诸暴强直, 皆属于风。"《灵枢·经筋》篇也说: "经筋之病, 寒则反折筋急。"《金匮要略》在继承《内经》理论的基础上, 不仅以表实无汗和表虚有汗分为刚痉、柔痉, 并提出了误治致痉的理论, 即表证过汗, 风病误下, 疮家误汗以及产后血虚, 汗出中风等, 致使外邪侵袭, 津液受伤, 筋脉失养, 而引发本证。《金匮要略》有关伤亡津液因而致痉的认识, 不仅对《内经》理论的发挥, 同时也为历代医家提供了内伤致痉的理论基础。《景岳全书·痉证》篇说: "凡属阴虚血少之辈, 不能养营筋脉, 以致搐挛僵仆者, 皆是此证。如中风之有此者, 必以年力衰残, 阴之败也; 产妇之有此者, 必以去血过多, 冲任竭也; 疮家之有此者, 必以血随脓出, 营气涸也; ……凡此之类, 总属阴虚之证。"温病学说的发展和成熟, 更进一步丰富和扩充了痉证病因病机的认识。提出了热盛伤津, 肝风内动, 引发本证的论述, 使痉证病因学说, 渐臻完备。如《温热经纬·薛生白湿热病篇》说: "木旺由于水亏, 故得引火生风, 反焚其本, 以致痉厥。"同时, 在外邪致痉中也补充了"湿热侵入经络脉髓中"的认识。

在中医学里尚有"瘈疭"一证。瘈疭即抽搐。《张氏医通·瘈疭》篇说: "瘈者, 筋脉拘急也, 疭者, 筋脉弛纵也, 俗谓之抽"。《温病条辨·痉病瘈疭总论》中又说: "痉者, 强直之谓, 后人所谓角弓反张, 古人所谓痉也。瘈者, 蠕动引缩之谓, 后人所谓抽掣, 搐搦, 古人所谓瘈也。"可见瘈疭即可为痉证症状表现之一, 也可单独出现而为病。

此外, 如因金疮破伤, 创口不洁, 感受风毒之邪, 也可发痉, 名为"破伤风"。因与一般痉证不尽相同, 故在外科加以介绍。

病因病机

痉证的病因病机, 归纳起来, 可分为外感和内伤两个方面。外感是风寒湿邪, 侵袭人体, 壅阻经络, 气血不畅, 或热盛动风, 或热灼津液而致痉。内伤是阴虚血少, 虚风内动, 筋脉失养而致痉。外感和内伤在病因上虽不相同, 但导致发痉的病机, 都是阴阳失调, 阳动而阴不濡所致。现分述如下:

(1) 邪壅经络　风寒湿邪, 壅滞脉络, 气血运行不利, 筋脉失养, 拘急而成痉。如《金匮要略方论本义·痉病总论》就痉证形成指出: "脉者人之正气正血所行之道路也, 杂错乎邪风、邪湿、邪寒, 则脉行之道路必阻塞壅滞, 而拘急蹉挛之证见矣。"

(2) 热甚发痉　热甚于里, 消灼津液, 阴液被伤, 筋脉失于濡养, 引起痉证, 或热病伤阴, 邪热内传营血, 热盛动风, 引发本证。如《临证指南医案·痉厥》篇所说: "五液劫尽, 阳气与内风鸱张, 遂变为痉"。

(3) 阴血亏损　素体阴虚血虚, 或因亡血, 或因汗下太过, 致使阴血损伤, 难以濡养筋脉, 因而成痉。正如《景岳全书·痉证》篇说: "凡属阴虚血少之辈, 不能养营筋脉, 以致搐挛僵仆

36　痉　　证

[215]

者。"

　　总之，痉证为筋脉之病。筋脉因风寒湿邪壅阻经络，气血不畅，失其濡养，或高热耗阴、亡血、过汗、误下等阴血亏竭，失其濡养，则筋脉拘急，而成痉证。正如《景岳全书·痉证》篇说："愚谓痉之为病，……其病在筋脉，筋脉拘急所以反张。"

　　类证鉴别

　　痉证应与中风、痫证作如下鉴别：

　　中风：中风可兼有筋脉拘急的抽搐症状，但同时可见口眼喎斜，半身不遂，清醒后多有后遗证。

　　痫证：昏迷时筋脉拘急，四肢抽搐，但为时较短，多吐涎沫，或发出异常叫声，苏醒抽搐即止，一如常人。

　　痉证：是以项背强直，四肢抽搐，甚则角弓反张为主症的病证，并可见于多种疾病的过程中。

　　辨证论治

　　本病临床以项背强急、四肢抽搐，甚至角弓反张为主症。临证宜详辨外感、内伤及其虚实。外感属实，内伤多虚。治实当祛邪，宜祛风、散寒、除湿、清热；治虚当扶正，宜滋阴养血，熄风舒筋通络。

　　（1）邪壅经络

　　〔症状〕　头痛，项背强直，恶寒发热，肢体酸重，苔白腻，脉浮紧。

　　〔证候分析〕　风寒湿邪，阻滞经络，故头痛，项背强直。外邪侵于肌表，营卫不和，则恶寒发热。湿阻经络肌肉，故肢体酸重。苔白腻，脉浮紧，均属风寒湿邪在表之候。

　　〔治法〕　祛风散寒，和营燥湿。

　　〔方药〕　羌活胜湿汤[213]。方中以羌活、独活、防风、藁本祛风胜湿；川芎、蔓荆子通络祛风止痛。邪祛络通，则痉自解。如寒邪较甚，苔薄白，脉浮紧，病属刚痉，治宜解肌发汗，方用葛根汤[347]治之。方中葛根解肌养筋，以舒拘急；麻黄、桂枝解表散寒；芍药、甘草益阴和里，并制麻桂发汗之猛；姜、枣调和营卫。如风邪偏盛，症见项背强直，发热不恶寒，头痛汗出，苔薄白，脉沉细，病属柔痉，治宜和营养津，方用栝蒌桂枝汤[275]。以桂枝汤调和营卫，解散表邪；栝蒌根清热生津，柔和筋脉。

　　若身热，筋脉拘急，胸脘痞闷，渴不欲饮，小便短赤，苔黄腻，脉滑数，此为湿热入络。治宜清热化湿，疏通经络，方用三仁汤[20]加地龙、秦艽、丝瓜络、威灵仙等以通经活络。

　　（2）热甚发痉

　　〔症状〕　发热胸闷，口噤齘齿，项背强直，甚至角弓反张，手足挛急，腹胀便秘，咽干口渴，心烦急躁，甚则神昏谵语，苔黄腻，脉弦数。

　　〔证候分析〕　邪热薰蒸阳明气分，宿滞中焦，阳明燥热内结，腑气不通，故胸闷、腹胀、便秘。热盛伤津，筋脉失养，则口噤齘齿，项背强直，甚至角弓反张，手足挛急，咽干口渴。热扰神明故心烦急躁，甚则神昏谵语。苔黄腻，脉弦数均为实热壅盛之象。

　　〔治法〕　泄热存津，养阴增液

　　〔方药〕　增液承气汤[381]。方中以大黄荡涤积热，芒硝软坚化燥；玄参、生地、麦冬养阴增液，滋润肠燥。使热去津回则热痉可解。如热盛伤津，并无腑实之证，可用白虎加人参汤[121]以清热救津。如抽搐较甚者，可酌加地龙、全蝎、菊花、钩藤等熄风通络之品。如烦躁较甚,可加淡竹叶,栀子清心除烦。

若温病邪热,内传营血,热盛动风,症见壮热头痛,神志昏迷,口噤抽搐,角弓反张,舌质红绛,苔黄燥,脉弦数,治以凉肝熄风,清热透窍。方用羚羊钩藤汤[333]。方中以羚羊角、钩藤、菊花、桑叶清热凉肝,熄风止痉;白芍、生地、甘草养阴增液,柔肝舒筋; 贝母、竹茹清热化痰;茯神宁心安神。神昏谵语或神志昏迷,可加服安宫牛黄丸[151]或至宝丹[148]以清热透窍。若邪热羁久,灼伤真阴,症见时时发痉,舌干少苔,脉虚数,可用大定风珠[28]以平肝熄风,养阴止痉。以上证治,同时可参照温病有关病证。

（3）阴血亏虚

[症状]　素体阴亏血虚,或在失血、汗、下太过之后,项背强急,四肢抽搐,头目昏眩,自汗,神疲,气短,舌淡红,脉弦细。

[证候分析]　气血两虚,不能营养筋脉,故项背强急,四肢抽搐。血虚不能上奉于脑,则头目昏眩。血去而元气耗伤, 卫外不固,故神疲气短而自汗。舌淡红,脉弦细均为阴血亏虚之征。

[治法]　滋阴养血

[方药]　四物汤[110]合大定风珠[28]加减。方中当归、川芎、白芍、熟地补血调血, 充养百脉。大定风珠平肝熄风, 养阴止痉。阴血得复,筋脉柔和,则痉证自除。如头晕、虚烦、失眠者,可加炒栀子、淡竹叶、菊花、夜交藤以清热安神,如纳呆腹满者,可加砂仁、鸡内金、陈皮等以理气和胃,如大便溏薄,面色㿠白,舌质淡,脉细者,可加党参、白术等以益气健脾。

结语

痉证是以阴阳失调, 阳动阴不濡而筋脉失养为主要病机的病证,其治疗,必须详辨外感与内伤,虚证与实证,切勿滥用镇潜熄风之品,治标而忽视其本。一般说, 外感发痉,多属实证,为外邪壅阻经络,气血运行不畅,或邪入里,热盛动风,或热灼津液,筋脉失养而成。邪盛者,先祛其邪,如属风寒湿邪,应分清主次,治宜祛风、散寒、除湿; 如邪热入里,实热内结,消灼阴液致痉者,治宜泄热存阴。内伤发痉,多属虚证,是由阴血不足,筋脉失养,肝风鼓动所致。正虚者,当先扶正。治宜滋阴养血。痉证在临床上属于阴伤血少者为多见,所以在治疗上滋养营阴是不可忽视的一环。

由于痉证往往多见于某些疾病的危重阶段,可危及生命,因此其防治颇为重要。见到高热、失血的病症,要及时清热、滋阴、养血,防止痉证的发生。

文献摘录

《灵枢·经筋》:"足少阴之筋,……其病……主痫瘈及痉,……在外者不能俯, 在内者不能仰,故阳病者,腰反折不能俯,阴病者不能仰。"

《素问·骨空论篇》:"督脉为病,脊强反折。"

《金匮要略·痉湿暍病》:"太阳病,发热无汗,反恶寒者,名曰刚痉。""太阳病,发热汗出,而不恶寒,名曰柔痉。""太阳病,其证备,身体强,几几然,脉反沉迟, 此为痉,栝蒌桂枝汤主之。""太阳病,无汗而小便反少,气上冲胸,口噤不得语,欲作刚痉,葛根汤主之。""痉为病,胸满口噤,卧不着席,脚挛急,必齘齿,可与大承气汤。"

《景岳全书·痉证》:"愚谓痉之为病,强直反张病也。其病在筋脉,筋脉拘急,所以反张。其病在血液,血液枯燥,所以筋挛。""痓之为病,即《内经》之痉病也,以痉作痓,盖传写之误耳。其证则脊背反张,头摇口噤,戴眼项强,四肢拘急,或见身热足寒,恶寒面赤之类皆是也。"

86 痉　　　证　　　　　　　　　　　　　　　[217]

《温热经纬·薛生白湿热病篇》:"湿热证,三四日即口噤,四肢牵引拘急,甚则角弓反张,此湿热侵入经络脉隧中, 宜鲜地龙、秦艽、威灵仙、滑石、苍耳子、丝瓜、海风藤、酒炒黄连等味。"

***Zhong Guo Zhen Jiu* (*Chinese Acupuncture & Moxibustion*) #5, 1994**
The Acupuncture Treatment of 34 Cases of (Skin) Chapping

针 刺 治 疗 皲 裂 34 例

全玳红　　王连芝
(中国刑警学院卫生所,沈阳110035)

1　一般资料

本组男性24例, 女性10例;年 龄 最小 30岁, 最大者50岁;病程在 2～10余年。治疗原则为调理气机、养阴润燥。

2　治疗方法

取患侧曲池、外关透内关、合谷透少府、足三里、三阴交。操作方法:选28号2.5～3寸毫针直刺, 用泻法;进针得气后留针10～15分钟, 每日针 1 次, 10次为 1 个疗程。

3　疗效标准

痊愈:经针刺 1 个疗程后, 手脚裂口愈合, 皮肤恢复正常, 1 年内不复发。

显效:经针刺 1 个疗程后手脚干燥明显好转, 裂口基本愈合, 1 年内复发 1 次。

好转:针刺后手脚干燥好转, 裂口有缩小。

无效:治疗前后的症状无变化。

4　治疗效果

本组34例大多经治疗 1 个疗程基本治愈, 有少数病例 2～3 年后复发。其中痊愈占79.4%, 显效占14.7%, 有效占2.9%, 无 效为 3 %, 总有效率为97%。

5　典型病例

刘××, 男, 45岁, 干部, 1985年 3 月来诊。自诉手足干裂, 久治不愈且反复发作已10年, 一年四季均有干裂尤 以 春、秋、冬 季 为重。按前法针灸后第 1 次冷汗出, 第 2 次手脚红润出汗, 3～4 次后干燥好转, 5～7 次后裂口基本愈合, 再针 5 次巩固疗效, 痊愈后随访 8 年未复发。

6　体会

祖国医学认为皮肤干裂、疼多为燥邪不敛肃降之气、耗伤人体津液后造成阴津亏虚, 如毛发不荣, 皮肤皲裂、大便秘结等。故刘宪素《素问玄机原病式》说:"诸涩枯涸干劲皲揭, 皆属于燥。"由于阴津亏虚, 肺不能肃降则引起气滞血瘀而等致皮肤干裂少汗、末稍血液循环障碍。

运用此法, 在于调整肃降、行气导滞, 气行则血行, 从而达到补阴生津、改 善 经 络 循行、使汗液分泌通畅, 减少瘀滞, 使手脚干燥得到改善, 皲裂的口子也就随之愈合。

(收稿日期: 1994-01-16)

Zhong Guo Zhen Jiu (*Chinese Acupuncture & Moxibustion*) #5, 1994, p. 24
Acupuncture plus Point Injection Therapy for 26 Cases of Trigeminal Neuralgia

针刺加穴位注射治疗三叉神经痛26例

韩小霞　钱轶显

（中国中医研究院针灸研究所，北京100700）

西医临床上治疗三叉神经痛多采用镇痛剂、射频热凝治疗、封闭或手术治疗等方法；中医除中药疗法外，运用针灸治疗亦很普遍，除单纯针刺疗法外，还有穴位激光照射、电针、穴位注射等疗法。据文献报道，运用穴位注射疗法有选用普鲁卡因及当归注射液者。我们所观察的病人是选用针刺加穴位注射野木瓜针剂，共治疗26例，取得了比较好的效果。

1　一般情况

本组26例中男10例，女16例；年龄最小33岁，最大76岁；病程最短3个月，最长20余年。

2　治疗方法

针刺加穴位注射野木瓜针剂，隔日治疗1次，10次为1疗程。

常用穴位：下关、风池、耳前、阿是穴（扳机点）。

以三叉神经第1支痛为主时加阳白、太阳、攒竹；第2支痛为主时加四白、颧髎、迎香、禾髎；第3支痛为主时加颊车、承浆、地仓等。均取患侧穴位。留针30分钟后起针，用2ml野木瓜注射液分2～3个穴位注射。

3　疗效观察

疗效评定主要是近期疗效，未作远期疗效的随访。近期疗效分：显效（疼痛明显缓解、停服一切镇痛剂，无自发性疼痛，偶有诱发性疼痛），进步（疼痛仍有发作，但其发作的程度、频率及持续时间均较治前减轻，镇痛剂服量亦减少），无效（病情无改善，镇痛剂服量如故）。

本组26例经针刺加穴位注射野木瓜针剂治疗后，显效19例，进步6例，无效1例。有效率为96.1%。其中疗程最短2次，最长25次。

4　典型病例

张××，男，58岁，工人。初诊：1993年11月6日。主诉：左侧面部阵发性疼痛1周。病史：患者于8年前1次煤气中毒后发生左侧面部阵发性疼痛，诊断为"三叉神经痛"。当时经单纯针刺治疗40余次后痊愈。此次就诊前1周因生气再次复发，每日凌晨4～5时发作，需服用2～4片去痛片方可缓解。经查疼痛区域位于三叉神经第2支分布区。行针刺左侧面部：下关、颧髎、地仓、颊车、风池穴，留针30分钟起针后，用野木瓜针剂2ml注射2个穴位，隔日治疗1次，经治6次后疼痛明显缓解，停服一切镇痛剂。

5　结论

三叉神经痛发病原因十分复杂。西医分为原发性三叉神经痛和继发性三叉神经痛两大类对其病因的认识有：血管压迫、机械压迫、病灶感染、中枢病原、缺血及病毒感染等学说。其共同病理机制为：半月神经节及神经根有退行性变，神经节细胞浆中出现空泡，神经纤维有退行性过度髓化及分节段性脱髓鞘伴轴索裸露的改变。中医将三叉神经痛归属为"头痛"、"偏头风"、"面痛"的范畴，其病因病机多为：风热或风寒挟痰阻络、肝郁化火及气虚血瘀等。由于痰湿瘀血阻滞经络引起经气不通导致疼痛。而野木瓜之药性具有祛风利湿、通经止痛之功，其用于穴位注射可使药效集中作用于神经周围以加强针刺镇痛之力，达到疏经活络、痛消病除之目的。

（收稿日期：1994-03-31）

Zhong Guo Zhen Jiu (***Chinese Acupuncture & Moxibustion***) **#4, 1994, p. 31**
A Depression Case History

郁证医案

谢×，男,11岁,学生。1991年11月9日晚7时许来诊。

其父代诉：患儿下午放学回家后集中精力在家做功课，因课外作业多而且有几道题做不出来，心里很着急，显得不耐烦，母亲就骂了他几句,过了几分钟，只见他悲伤欲哭，叹大气，继而哭笑不止，时有喃喃自语，家人怎么安慰和经手法按摩都不能制止而前来就诊。查体：见悲伤啼哭而不能发泄，哭笑交作，多语。问及头晕，怕冷。神志清楚，对答正常。舌淡红，苔薄白，脉弦有力。

诊断：郁证，证属郁怒不畅，心神失常。治疗，拟疏肝解郁，养心安神。取双侧行间、神门，行间施泻法，神门平补平泻。针刺得气后其大哭少笑，留针20分钟拔针。哭笑停止，诉轻度头晕，观察10分钟诸症消失如常人而归。随访至今未发生过类似病症。

**按语：此例病人先有思虑过度，加之家长的训骂，使之情志受伤，郁怒不畅，肝失条达，扰乱心神。治则遵《素问·六元正纪大论》指出："木郁达之"。取行间疏肝解郁，神门开心窍以苏神明。

341100　江西省赣县人民医院　　曾建亚

（收稿日期：1992-12-10）

Zhong Guo Zhen Jiu (***Chinese Acupuncture & Moxibustion***) **#5, 1994, p. 194**
A Survey of the Treatment Efficacy of 116 Cases of One-sided Wind Stroke Paralysis
Treated by Acupuncture-Moxibustion

针灸治疗中风偏瘫116例疗效观察

张　秀　芳
（甘肃省张掖市人民医院，734000）

1　临床资料

116例患者，男性91例，女性25例；年龄最小23岁，最大85岁，平均年龄为54岁；病程短的2天，最长的2年，多数在半年之内。

2　治疗方法

中经络（半身不遂）：调和经脉，疏通气血，取穴以阳明经穴为主，辅以膀胱经、胆经穴位。取患侧，头部：百会、太阳、风池；上肢：肩髃、曲池、外关、合谷、后溪；下肢：环跳、委中、足三里、阳陵泉、昆仑。中枢性面瘫加地仓、颊车，失语加廉泉，有阴虚阳亢证者泻太冲、补太溪，气血虚者补足三里。痰湿盛者取丰隆。

中脏腑闭证，取督脉和十二井穴为主，用毫针泻法或三棱针点刺出血。取穴：人中、十二井穴、太冲、丰隆、劳宫。脱症取任脉经穴为主，取关元、神阙，大艾炷隔盐灸。

用28～30号毫针。平补平泻（初病宜泻，久病宜补）手法针刺，每次30～40分钟。配合G6805型治疗仪断续波30分钟后，艾条在针刺穴位上施灸10～15分钟。每日上下肢交替针刺。治疗过程中，叮嘱患者活动肢体，并让患者家属早晚搓上下肢体，起按摩作用，促进血液循环。四周为一疗程，每疗程间隔一周。

3　疗效标准

痊愈：言语正常，上肢能高举握物、解衣扣、拧瓶盖，下肢能独立行走，生活自理，恢复工作者。

显效：上肢握物无力，下肢独立行走，言语能表达意思。

好转：语言不清或上下肢功能明显好转，尤其下肢扶杖可行短距离者。

无效：虽有进步或中断治疗者。

4　治疗结果

本组痊愈54例，占46.55%，显效34例，占29.31%；好转28例，占24.14%。有效率为100.00%。

（收稿日期：1993-06-08）

Ming Yi Ming Fang Lu (A Record of Famous Doctor's Famous Formulas)
Jia Wei Wu Bei Ji Gan San (Added Flavors Sepia, Fritillaria, Bletilla, & Licorice Powder)

加味乌贝芨甘散

组成　三七粉 30 克　乌贼骨 30 克　川贝 30 克
白芨 30 克　黄连 30 克　甘草 30 克
砂仁 15 克　延胡索 30 克　川楝肉 30 克
佛手 30 克　广木香 18 克　生白芍 45 克

用法　共研为极细末，每日早、中、晚饭后各吞 3 克，连续服用 3 个月至半年。

功能　柔肝和胃，调气活血，制酸止痛，止血生肌。

主治　胃溃疡、十二指肠溃疡病（肝胃不和）、胃脘痛、泛酸、呕吐、便黑、呕血等症。

方解　本方以三七粉为主药，能止血、散血、定痛，亦主呕血、下血；乌贼骨收敛制酸，止痛止血；川贝化瘀，散结消肿，与乌贼骨配伍有较强的制酸止痛作用。白芨收敛止血，消肿生肌；芍药、甘草酸甘化阴，柔肝缓急止痛；黄连清热燥湿，川楝肉、延胡索、佛手、广木香行气活血止痛，砂仁理气健脾，合而具柔肝和胃、调气活血之功。为散，便于常服，缓攻徐图，促进溃疡愈合，以期根治。本方亦可据证作适当加减。

典型病例　某女，18 岁，脘痛 2 年余。自述脘痛阵作，入夜加重，辗转难眠，上腹及两胁胀满，时有反酸，嗳气频频，苔薄白，脉弦。经 X 光钡餐检查，见十二指肠球部有 1×1.3cm 龛影，诊断为十二指肠球部溃疡。本病例肝胃不和，气滞较甚，于散中加入制香附 18 克，以增强疏肝理气、和胃止痛之力，嘱其早、中、晚饭后各服 3 克，坚持服用三月，诸症好转。X 线钡餐复查，十二指肠球部龛影消失痊愈，至今已 17 年未复发。

Zhong Guo Zhen Jiu (Chinese Acupuncture & Moxibustion) #5, 1994
The Acupuncture-Moxibustion Treatment of 32 Cases of Adolescent Neurasthenia

针刺治疗儿童抽动秽语综合征32例

张 开 权
（四川省内江市第一人民医院针灸科，641000）

儿童抽动秽语综合征是指儿童的一种突然发生、重复或交替出现的不随意运动，以面部或颈部多组肌肉抽动及不自主发声为其特点。笔者自1990年来采用针刺治疗本病32例，取得较满意疗效，现总结如下。

1 临床资料

本组32例均经门诊检查除外器质性病变，其中男性29例，女性3例；年龄最小5岁，最大11岁；病程最短10天，最长为6个月。其中有21例经用药物治疗无显著效果而来针治。

2 治疗方法

2.1 取穴：大椎、风池、合谷。局部配穴：眨眼、耸鼻加太阳、迎香；口角抽动加地仓、颊车。局部均取患侧，交替使用。

2.2 操作：穴位局部皮肤用75％酒精常规消毒，选用28号1寸毫针，快速进针，捻转时手法要轻，平补平泻，得气后留针20分钟，每日1次，7次为1疗程、中间休息2～3天。

3 疗效标准

痊愈：抽动完全消失，运动功能恢复正常。

显效：抽动程度明显减轻，各症状缓解。

无效：治疗前后症状无明显改变。

4 治疗结果

本组32例患儿中痊愈24例，占75.0％；显效7例，占21.9％；无效1例，占3.1％。有效率96.7％。

5 典型病例

康×，男，6岁。其母代诉，患儿近20天来经常不自主的挤眉眨眼，左肩关节也频繁抽动，睡觉时症状消失，经服用药物治疗无效而前来针灸。按上法取穴治疗，2次后，患儿抽动程度明显减轻；治疗1个疗程后诸症消失而告痊愈。半年后随访未见复发。

6 体会

本病的发生主要由于儿童时期"稚阳未充"、"稚阴未长"，各组织器官神经功能发育尚未成熟，营卫失调，卫外不固，风邪乘虚而入或气血虚弱、经脉失养所致。治疗当疏散风邪、调和营卫为主。大椎为手足三阳经与督脉之交会，最善调节经络气机逆乱，为通络解痉之要穴；风池乃手足少阳与阳维之会，既疏散外风，又平熄内风，内外兼治；合谷系手阳明经原穴，贯频经面部和足阳明相联系。根据"经脉所过，主治所及"和阳明经多气多血的原理。针刺此三穴可获调和营卫、疏风活络兼益气血之效应，解除抽动肌肉的痉挛状态，而达到治疗目的。

针刺治疗本病，取穴少、疗程短、见效快，又无任何不良反应，病人易接受，便于推广。

（收稿日期：1994-03-14）

Ming Yi Ming Fang Lu (*A Record of Famous Doctor's Famous Formulas*)
Ya Tong De Xiao Fang (Toothache Get Effect Formula) p. 296

牙痛得效方

组成　生地 15～30 克　淮山药 15 克　杭萸肉 6 克
　　　　云苓 10 克　泽泻 10 克　丹皮 12 克
　　　　丹参 30 克　骨碎补 15 克　银花 12 克

功能　养肾清肾固齿　滋阴降火。

主治　各种牙痛。

用法　每日 1 剂,早晚各 1 煎,食后服。

方解　本方根据肾主骨、牙为骨之余、治牙痛以治肾为主的理论,选用六味地黄丸加减而成。方中六味地黄丸养肾清肾固齿,滋阴降火以治其本。加骨碎补入肾入骨,补肾补伤,治风血疼痛,养筋络,固精髓,疗齿痛,为治牙痛之要药;丹参活血,治寒热积聚;银花解毒清热,治风火牙痛。

加减运用　兼有外感风热之邪者,重用银花,加连翘、知母、生石膏;若因风寒之邪客于牙体,致牙齿疼痛,患牙得热则痛减者,去银花,加麻黄、细辛、清半夏。

禁忌　服药期间应忌烟、酒、辛辣等对口腔有刺激的食物。

按语　牙痛是一种常见病、多发病,虽然不至于危及生命,却也是"痛起来要命"。临床上以风火牙痛和虚火牙痛为多。上方是治疗牙痛的基本方,牙为骨之余,肾之所主。牙之为病,必为肾之失司,临证必以治肾固齿为要,随邪之所禀,辨证加减。

抓住主证,整体调治,陈氏学术思想,可见一斑

Ming Yi Ming Fang Lu (*A Record of Famous Doctor's Famous Formulas*)
Bu Wei Jiang Ya Tang (Eight Flavors Downbear Pressure Decoction) p. 338-339

八味降压汤

组成　何首乌 15 克　白芍 12 克　当归 9 克
　　　　川芎 5 克　炒杜仲 18 克　黄芪 30 克
　　　　黄柏 6 克　钩藤 30 克

功能　益气养血,滋阴泻火。

主治　凡表现为阴血亏虚、头痛、眩晕、神疲乏力,耳鸣心悸等症的原发性高血压病、肾性高血压以及更年期综合征、心脏神经官能症等,均可用本方治疗。

用法　先将药物用适量水浸泡 1 小时左右,煎两次,首煎 10～15 分钟,以保留药物的易挥发成分;二煎 30～50 分钟,文火。煎好后将两煎混合,总量约 250～300 毫升,每日 1 剂,每剂分 2～3 次服用,饭后 2 小时左右温服。

方解　高血压病的病因不一，发展到一定程度，其基本病机是阴阳失调，营血亏虚，血行不畅。因而方用首乌、白芍、杜仲养其阴血；芎、归行其血滞；阴血的滋润有赖于阳气的温煦，故用黄芪益气配阳以助阴；"阴虚而阳盛，先补其阴，而后泻其阳以和之"，黄柏、钩藤之用意就在于此。全方合伍，使肾有所滋，脑有所养，肝有所平，从而达到血养风熄、血压得降的目的。

加减运用　伴失眠、烦躁者，加炒枣仁 30 克、夜交藤 30 克、栀子 9 克；便稀苔腻、手足肿胀者，加半夏 9 克、白术 12 克、泽泻 30 克；大便干燥加生地 30 克、仙灵脾 18 克；上热下寒、舌红口干、面热、足冷，加黄连 5 克、肉桂 5 克。

方歌　八味乌芍与归芎，钩藤芪柏炒杜仲；
　　　　　阴血亏虚高血压，加减变应服之平。

按语　本方系根据日人大塚敬节之经验方"八物降下汤"化裁而来。

论文摘要　高血压病的发生发展变化，从中医的角度来看，不外肝的气血失和，脾的升降失司，肾的阴阳失调。就一般情况而言，高血压病初期大多始于肝，进而影响脾，最后归结于肾，形成肾阴不足、肝阳上亢的高血压病。本病之头痛、眩晕、心悸、脉弦等阳亢的实证为标象，而阴血亏虚为本质。血压增高的实质，是由器官供血不足而造成的。动脉血压的维持，原是为了"血主濡之，以奉生身"，保证体内各个器官正常血液的供求平衡，尤其心、脑、肾最为重要。治疗高血压病不能单纯求之降压药物，用时则降，停药则升，首先要供给重要器官所需的气血，才能达到降压的目的，即所谓"欲夺之，先予之"。使周身气血"升已而降，降已而升"，有规律地运行不息，达到"阴平阳秘"的动态平衡，血压才能稳定于正常范围。多年的临床实践证明，八味降压汤就能起到这种作用，从而取得显著的疗效。

Appendix 3:
More Exercises for Practicing Writing Characters

新		xīn
干		gān
净		jìng
复		fù
预		yù
看		kàn
说		shuō
听		tīng
录		lù
音		yīn
晚		wǎn
上		shàng
课		kè
练		liàn
同		tóng
问		wèn

今									jīn
天									tiān
去									qù
儿									ér
安									ān
门									mén
怎									zěn
样									yàng

学									xué
习									xí
什									shén
么									me
汉									hàn
语									yǔ
也									yě
我									wǒ

正视接话复闻表团观厂访照片打明城玩出发

Appendix 4:
Different Styles of Chinese Typefaces

Just as in English, there are many different typefaces used to print Chinese. The following is a list of a number of titles of the articles in the *Si Chuan Zhong Yi* (*Sichuan Chinese Medicine*), #1, 1998. As you can see, these titles are printed in a number of different fonts or faces. Some are *kai shu*, some are *song shu*, some are *li shu*, and some are *xing shu*. In addition, there are analogs of what we would call serifed and sans-serifed faces as well as ornamental or decorative faces. See if you can translate all of these. The *xing shu* will be the hardest. Happily, the table of contents in the front of the journal uses a very simple *kai shu* face. So you can always translate the table of contents title even if you can't read the fancy title on the first page of the article.

顾伯华教授治疗乳癖的经验

足跟部滑囊炎治验

针刺治疗血管性头痛 42 例

全体重导引术颈牵治疗神经根型颈椎病 228 例临床报告

电针加 TDP 照射治疗女性尿道综合征 42 例

中西医结合治疗血栓闭塞性脉管炎 37 例

罕见病治验二则

柴胡龙牡汤治疗老年性室性早搏

徐福松男科杂症牵隅

黄芪苁蓉煎治虚秘 40 例临床观察

大承气汤治疗胃大部切除术后排空障碍的疗效观察

以虫类药为基础治疗脑梗塞 60 例

内外并治缓解期慢性支气管炎哮喘

青蒿鳖甲汤加味治疗顽固性高热举隅

膈下逐瘀汤治疗前列腺增生 22 例

李达祥内病外治验案三则

黄芪地龙汤治疗慢性乳糜尿 45 例

中医治疗胃脘痛顽症 96 例

中药注射液治疗脑梗塞 28 例

加味金刚丸治疗格林－巴利综合征 7 例

FIRE IN THE VALLEY: TCM Diagnosis & Treatment of Vaginal Diseases ISBN 0-936185-25-2

FLESHING OUT THE BONES: The Importance of Case Histories in Chin. Med. trans. by Chip Chace. ISBN 0-936185-30-9

FU QING-ZHU'S GYNECOLOGY trans. by Yang Shou-zhong and Liu Da-wei, ISBN 0-936185-35-X

FULFILLING THE ESSENCE: A *Handbook of Traditional & Contemporary Treatments for Female Infertility* by Bob Flaws, ISBN 0-936185-48-1

GOLDEN NEEDLE WANG LE-TING: A 20th Century Master's Approach to Acupuncture by Yu Hui-chan and Han Fu-ru, trans. by Shuai Xue-zhong,

A HANDBOOK OF TRADITIONAL CHINESE D-ERMATOLOGY by Liang Jian-hui, trans. by Zhang & Flaws, ISBN 0-936185-07-4

A HANDBOOK OF TRADITIONAL CHINESE G-YNECOLOGY by Zhejiang College of TCM, trans. by Zhang Ting-liang, ISBN 0-936185-06-6 (4th edit.)

A HANDBOOK OF MENSTRUAL DISEASES IN CHINESE MEDICINE by Bob Flaws ISBN 0-936185-82-1

A HANDBOOK of TCM PEDIATRICS by Bob Flaws, ISBN 0-936185-72-4

A HANDBOOK OF TCM UROLOGY & MALE SEXUAL DYSFUNCTION by Anna Lin, OMD, ISBN 0-936185-36-8

THE HEART & ESSENCE OF DAN-XI'S METH-ODS OF TREATMENT by Xu Dan-xi, trans. by Yang, ISBN 0-926185-49-X

THE HEART TRANSMISSION OF MEDICINE by Liu Yi-ren, trans. by Yang Shou-zhong ISBN 0-936185-83-X

HIGHLIGHTS OF ANCIENT ACUPUNCTURE PRESCRIPTIONS trans. by Wolfe & Crescenz ISBN 0-936185-23-6

How to Have A HEALTHY PREGNANCY, HEAL-THY BIRTH with Chinese Medicine by Honora Lee Wolfe, ISBN 0-936185-40-6

HOW TO WRITE A TCM HERBAL FORMULA: *A Logical Methodology for the Formulation & Administration of Chinese Herbal Medicine in Decoction* by Bob Flaws, ISBN 0-936185-49-X

IMPERIAL SECRETS OF HEALTH & LONGEV-ITY by Bob Flaws, ISBN 0-936185-51-1

KEEPING YOUR CHILD HEALTHY WITH CHINESE MEDICINE by Bob Flaws, ISBN 0-936185-71-6

Li Dong-yuan's TREATISE ON THE SPLEEN & STOMACH, *A Translation of the Pi Wei Lun* by Yang Shou-zhong & Li Jian-yong, ISBN 0-936185-41-4

LOW BACK PAIN: Care & Prevention with Chin-ese Medicine by Douglas Frank, ISBN 0-936185-66-X

MASTER HUA'S CLASSIC OF THE CENTRAL VISCERA by Hua Tuo, ISBN 0-936185-43-0

THE MEDICAL I CHING: *Oracle of the Healer Within* by Miki Shima, OMD, ISBN 0-936185-38-4

MANAGING MENOPAUSE NATURALLY with Chinese Medicine by Honora Lee Wolfe ISBN 0-936185-98-8

PAO ZHI: Introduction to Processing Chinese Medicinals to Enhance Their Therapeutic Effect, by Philippe Sionneau, ISBN 0-936185-62-1

PATH OF PREGNANCY, VOL. I, Gestational Disorders by Bob Flaws, ISBN 0-936185-39-2

PATH OF PREGNANCY, Vol. II, Postpartum Diseases by Bob Flaws. ISBN 0-936185-42-2

PEDIATRIC BRONCHITIS: Its Cause, Diagnosis & Treatment According to TCM trans. by Gao Yu-li and Bob Flaws, ISBN 0-936185-26-0

PRINCE WEN HUI'S COOK: Chinese Dietary Therapy by Bob Flaws & Honora Lee Wolfe, ISBN 0-912111-05-4, $12.95 (Published by Paradigm Press)

THE PULSE CLASSIC: A Translation of the *Mai Jing* by Wang Shu-he, trans. by Yang Shou-zhong ISBN 0-936185-75-9

RECENT TCM RESEARCH FROM CHINA, trans. by Charles Chace & Bob Flaws, ISBN 0-936185-56-2

THE SECRET OF CHINESE PULSE DIAGNOSIS by Bob Flaws, ISBN 0-936185-67-8

SEVENTY ESSENTIAL TCM FORMULAS FOR BEGINNERS by Bob Flaws, ISBN 0-936185-59-7

SHAOLIN SECRET FORMULAS for Treatment of External Injuries, by De Chan, ISBN 0-936185-08-2

STATEMENTS OF FACT IN TRADITIONAL CHINESE MEDICINE by Bob Flaws, ISBN 0-936185-52-X